The health of indigenous people is an issue that too many governments have avoided and neglected for far too long with the result being that very many of the world's indigenous populations have health outcomes far inferior to majority populations. This book makes it clear that these unacceptable outcomes are politically and socially determined and seeks to locate indigenous health outcomes in a context of several decades of global market integration that has seen some better outcomes for some indigenous populations but which has also thrown up considerable inequalities that make improved health and lifestyles for these populations a vital challenge for policy makers and for the communities involved. Innovative responses are required, and this book provides the basis for far better informed approaches to indigenous health outcomes.

Kevin Hewison, Weldon E. Thornton Distinguished Emeritus Professor at the University of North Carolina at Chapel Hill

This book provides an impressive overview of the problems that continue to face indigenous peoples all over the developed and developing world. Variously marginalised by processes of modernisation, colonisation, industrial development and globalisation, those that can be defined as indigenous peoples almost everywhere face discrimination and are disproportionately represented in the ranks of the socially and economically disadvantaged. Such a situation, as the book shows, can be easily discerned from the generally poorer conditions of health that indigenous peoples generally enjoy. The book raises important questions about how we understand such fundamental issues as social justice, development and modernity on the basis of the plight of indigenous peoples.

Vedi Hadiz, Professor of Asian Studies at the University of Melbourne, Australia

This important contribution to indigenous studies highlights changes initiated by the forces of globalization. It is an extremely interesting study that weaves together stories of various indigenous groups across the world to discuss policy failures and ramifications.

Ahmed Shafiqul Huque, PhD, Professor and Chair, Department of Political Science, McMaster University, Canada

T0174730

Globalization and the Health of Indigenous Peoples

In 70 countries worldwide, there are an estimated 370 million Indigenous peoples, and their rich diversity of cultures, religions, traditions, languages and histories has been a significant source of our scholarships. However, the health status of this population group is far below that of non-Indigenous populations by all standards. Could the persisting reluctance to understand the influence of self-governance, globalization and social determinants of health in the lives of these people be deemed as a contributor to the poor health of Indigenous peoples?

Within this volume, Ullah explores the gap in health status between Indigenous and non-Indigenous peoples by providing a comparative assessment of socioeconomic and health indicators for Indigenous peoples, government policies, and the ways in which Indigenous peoples have been resisting and adapting to state policies.

A timely book for a growing field of study, *Globalization and the Health of Indigenous Peoples* is a must read for academics, policy makers, and practitioners who are interested in Indigenous studies and in understanding the role that globalization plays for the improvement of Indigenous peoples' health across the world.

AKM Ahsan Ullah is Associate Professor of Geography, Environment and Development studies and Deputy Dean of Graduate Studies and Research, Faculty of Arts and Social Sciences (FASS), at the University of Brunei Darussalam, Brunei.

Routledge Studies in Health and Social Welfare

For a full list of titles in this series, please visit www.routledge.com

Globalization and the Health of Indigenous Peoples

From Colonization to Self-Rule

AKM Ahsan Ullah

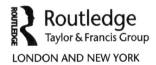 Routledge
Taylor & Francis Group

LONDON AND NEW YORK

First published 2017
by Routledge

2 Park Square, Milton Park, Abingdon, Oxfordshire OX14 4RN
52 Vanderbilt Avenue, New York, NY 10017

Routledge is an imprint of the Taylor & Francis Group, an informa business

First issued in paperback 2019

British Library Cataloguing in Publication Data
A catalogue record for this book is available from the British Library

Library of Congress Cataloging in Publication Data
A catalog record for this book has been requested

ISBN: 978-1-138-82187-3 (hbk)
ISBN: 978-0-367-86950-2 (pbk)

Typeset in Times New Roman
by Apex CoVantage, LLC

Contents

Illustrations

Figure

Tables

Map

Abbreviations

ABS	Australian Bureau of Statistics
ACOBOL	Female Councilors' Association of Bolivia
AIWN	Asian Indigenous Women's Network
ALMG	Academy of Maya Languages of Guatemala
AMAP	Arctic Monitoring and Assessment Programme
ANIPA	Plural National Indigenous Assembly for Autonomy
ATSIC	Aboriginal and Torres Strait Islander Commission
BBC	British Broadcasting Corporation
BCS	Bangladesh Civil Service
BNP	Bangladesh National Party
BRAC	Bangladesh Rural Advancement Committee
CDEP	Community Development Employment Projects
CDES	Centre for Economic and Social Rights
CEH	Commission for Historical Clarification
CEJIS	Center for Indigenous and Social Legal Studies
CHT	Chittagong Hill Tracts
CHTDF	Chittagong Hill Tracts Development Fund
CHTRC	Chittagong Hill Tracts Regional Council
CIHI	Canadian Institute for Health Information
CIP	Permanent Indian Congress
CIRABO	Bolivian Amazon Indigenous Coordinating Committee
CIT	Tayrona Indigenous Confederation
CNE	National Electoral Convention of Indigenous Peoples
CNI	National Indigenous Congress
CNN	Cable News Network
CNPI	National Council of Indigenous Peoples
COMG	Council of Mayan Organizations of Guatemala
COPMAGUA	Coordination of Organizations of the Mayan People of Guatemala
CPP	Communist Party of the Philippines
CRIC	Cauca Regional Indigenous Council
DIAND	Department of Indian Affairs and Northern Development
DUSAKAW	Indigenous Health Care Providing Enterprise in Northern Colombia

ECOSOC	United Nations Economic and Social Council
EMRIP	Expert Mechanism on the Rights of Indigenous Peoples
ESC	Economic and Social Council
EU	European Union
FIB	Indigenous Federation of the State of Bolivar
FPIC	Free, Prior and Informed Consent
GCG	Global Coordinating Group
HDC	Hill District Councils
HIV/AIDS	Human immunodeficiency virus infection / acquired immunodeficiency syndrome
HRC	Human Rights Council
HRDC	Human Resources Development Canada
HREOC	Human Rights and Equal Opportunity Commission
IASG	Inter-Agency Support Group
ICTs	Information and Communications Technologies
IDH	Human Development Rate
IDRC	International Development Research Centre
IFAD	International Fund for Agricultural Development
ILO	International Labor Organization
IOM	Organization of International Migrations
IPGREN	Indigenous Peoples' Global Research and Education Network
IPDs	Private Development Institutions
IWGIA	International Work Group for Indigenous Affairs
MDGs	Millennium Development Goals
MMP	Mixed Member Proportional
MoCHTA	Ministry of Chittagong Hill Tracts Affairs
MSRQ	Ministère de la Sécurité du revenu du Québec
NAFTA	North American Free Trade Agreement
NATSIHS	National Aboriginal and Torres Strait Islander Health Survey
NCCAH	National Collaborating Centre for Aboriginal Health
NGO	Nongovernmental Organization
NPE	New Economic Policy
NWAC	Native Women's Association of Canada
OAS	Organisation of American States
OAU	Organization of African Unity
OIA	Indigenous Organization of Antioquia
OIK	Kankuamo Indigenous Organization
OISE	Indigenous Organization of Ecuador
ONIC	National Indigenous Organization of Colombia
OSC	Civil Society Organizations
PCJSS	Parbatya Chattagram Jana Samhati Samiti
PEA	Economically Active Population
RC	Regional Council
RCAP	Royal Commission on Aboriginal Peoples
SDH	Social Determinants of Health

SPCPD	Southern Philippines Council for Peace and Development
SR	Special Rapporteur
SZOPAD	Special Zone for Peace and Development
TNC	Transnational Corporations
UN	United Nations
UNCED	United Nations Conference on Environment and Development
UNDP	United Nations Development Programme
UNDRIP	United Nations Declaration on the Rights of Indigenous Peoples
UNESCO	United Nations Educational, Scientific and Cultural Organization
UNFCCC	United Nations Framework Convention on Climate Change
UNGA	United Nations General Assembly
UNHCR	United Nations High Commissioner for Refugees
UNHRC	United Nations Human Rights Council
UNICEF	United Nations International Children's Emergency Fund
USAID	US Agency for International Development
WGIP	Working Group on Indigenous Populations
WHC	World Heritage Committee
WHO	World Health Organization
WIMSA	Working Group of Indigenous Minorities in Southern Africa
WIPO	World Intellectual Property Organization

1 Introduction

Indigenous Peoples in the Globalizing World

Indigenous peoples are considered to be the preservers of the diversity of the world. There is no doubt that they have been holding the world's linguistic and cultural diversity for centuries. According to the United Nations (2009), their traditional culture and knowledge have been a significant resource for humanity. This means that they demand an important space in the global discourse about belief systems, development and culture. Yet, they remain one of the most disadvantaged groups in the world. To varying degrees across the world, they are subject to discrimination and marginalization. There is evidence not only in developing countries but also in developed countries that they have been deprived of the rights to their traditional land (UN, 2009). This is one of the primary factors that is responsible for their longstanding condition of poverty. Indigenous peoples include a disproportionate percentage of the poor, the illiterate, and the unemployed people in the world. For example, Indigenous peoples constitute approximately 5 percent of the world's population; however, they make up 15 percent of the world's poor and about one-third of the world's 900 million extremely rural poor. They form about 5,000 distinct groups and occupy about 20 percent of the earth's territory (IFAD, 2007). However, due to degradation of their traditional land and eviction from their ancestral land, they have begun to move to urban areas. This is perhaps one of the most telling single measures of their inequitable access to the social determinants of health; one that is even more exacerbated by the negligence of authorities in most countries that rely on rights-based obligations for the assurance of their wellbeing.

The very existence of groups of people identified as 'Indigenous' is a result of earlier centuries of globalization. Without colonization of the 'new world' by Europeans, and the migrations of tribal groups throughout the world that characterized much of human history, there would not be people identified as having been first in a certain locale (David, 1997). This chapter may not concern itself with the effects on Indigenous peoples and their health during this earlier process of globalization, which has been well documented and often characterized by a bacterial or viral genocide, not always unintended. Rather, we are concerned with how the last 25 years of increased global market integration has created opportunities or barriers to Indigenous peoples' access to the social determinants of health (SDH), partly—though not solely—through increased potentials for economic self-determination, political self-rule and cultural regeneration.

This means the colonial legacy has had a long-term impact on their life. Their right to development has been largely denied by colonial and modern states in the pursuit of economic growth. As a consequence, Indigenous peoples often lose out to more powerful actors, becoming among the most impoverished groups in their respective countries (United Nations, 2009).

> "Before the plantation came in, our lifestyle was prosperous. If we needed fruits, we just went to the forest. It was the same if we needed medicines, we just went to the forest. But since this company came in and burned our forest, everything has gone. Our life became difficult. The forest fire has been a disaster for us"—a member of the Adat community, Indonesia.
> (Asian Development Bank, 2002 mentioned in UN, 2009)

This chapter begins with a brief consideration of what is meant by 'Indigenous' and some tabulation of where most of the world's Indigenous are located. It proceeds to a review of how globalization is affecting the SDH, with specific reference to Indigenous people. It concludes with consideration of the prospects of improved Indigenous health via improved SDH through increased self-governance. This chapter reviews the impact of contemporary globalization on the Indigenous population and eventually on health. It also examines how Indigenous populations and Indigenous people adopt different self-governance strategies to improve their health and what effect globalization has had on these efforts.

The Indigenous Population's Response

Defining *Indigenous* is complex. For the last four decades, the debate about the definition of *Indigenous* has been ongoing. However, so far no definition has been adopted by any organization, including the United Nations. Martínez-Cobo (1986: 7) offered a working definition of Indigenous communities, peoples and nations:

> Indigenous communities, peoples and nations are those which, having a historical continuity with pre-invasion and pre-colonial societies that developed on their territories, consider themselves distinct from other sectors of the societies now prevailing on those territories, or parts of them. They form at present non-dominant sectors of society and are determined to preserve, develop and transmit to future generations their ancestral territories, and their ethnic identity, as the basis of their continued existence as peoples, in accordance with their own cultural patterns, social institutions and legal system.

The concept of "Indigenous peoples" still remains contentious. No signs are seen for a resolution of the controversy in the near future. In an effort, the UN, the ILO and the World Bank offered three approaches to the definitional controversy.

There has been a working definition used by the 1986 report of UN Special Rapporteur, which is:

> Indigenous communities, peoples and nations are those which, having a historical continuity with pre-invasion and pre-colonial societies that developed on their territories, consider themselves distinct from other sectors of the societies now prevailing in those territories, or parts of them. They form at present non-dominant sectors of society and are determined to preserve, develop and transmit to future generations their ancestral territories, and their ethnic identity, as the basis of their continued existence as peoples, in accordance, with their own cultural patterns, social institutions and legal systems.

Like many other countries elsewhere, governments of major Asian states deny Indigenous rights. As a result, the attitudes of governments to the application within their states of the concept of "Indigenous peoples" differ considerably; however, opposition has been expressed by some countries, such as China, India, Bangladesh, Myanmar and Indonesia. The argument some governments of Asian states make is that the concept of "Indigenous peoples" is an outcome of the experience of European colonial settlement; therefore, it may not be applicable to those parts of Asia that did not experience European settlement (Erni, 2008). This denial presents multifaceted problems. This deters large number of Indigenous peoples in the region from participating in the Working Group's deliberations, resulting in withholding the benefits of the Declaration from the Indigenous, tribal, and Aboriginal peoples of Asia.

In defining the Indigenous, historical continuity of occupation of ancestral lands, common ancestry with the original occupants of these lands, culture in general, language (whether used as the only language, as mother tongue, as the habitual means of communication at home or in the family, or as the main, preferred, habitual, general or normal language), and residence in certain parts of the country or in certain regions in the world are considered significant factors.

The debates surrounding this definition will continue to remain because this definition is based on "historical continuity with pre-invasion and pre-colonial societies that developed on their territories" (Ferreira, 2013). The World Bank, however, has dispensed altogether with criteria based on historical continuity and colonialism, instead taking a functional view of "Indigenous peoples" as "groups with a social and cultural identity distinct from the dominant society that makes them vulnerable to being disadvantaged" (Erni, 2008). In answering who are the Indigenous peoples, Ferreira (2013: 8) explains:

> there are some fundamental criterion of self-identification of the Indigenous, which are: Self-identification as Indigenous Peoples at the individual level and acceptance as a member by the community; Historical continuity with pre-colonial and/or pre-settler societies; Strong link to territories and surrounding natural resources; Distinct social, economic, or political systems; Distinct language, culture, and knowledge; Status as a non-dominant social

group; Resolve to maintain and reproduce ancestral environments and systems as distinctive peoples and communities.

On an individual basis, an Indigenous person is one who belongs to these Indigenous populations through self-identification as Indigenous (group consciousness) and who is recognized and accepted by these populations as one of its members (acceptance by the group) (UN, 2009). Clearly, they practice a distinct social, cultural, economic and political life. According to the common definition, they are the descendants of those who inhabited the world, from the Arctic to the South Pacific, at the times when people of different cultures or ethnic origins arrived. The new arrivals later became dominant through conquest, occupation, settlement or other means (UN, 2010).

The majority (about 70 percent) of Indigenous people live in Asia. Hence, Asia is the most culturally diverse region in the world (IWGIA, 2012). However, these populations face more discrimination and marginalization than those in the West. Forced assimilation and encroachment of dominant groups into their own territories are the most common ordeals they face. While several countries have good legislation to protect the rights of Indigenous peoples, in most cases their rights are often violated and overruled. About 14 percent are in Africa (about 50 million). Still, most of them are nomadic and seminomadic pastoralists and hunters. Prior to the declaration of independence of Israel in 1948, around 90,000 Bedouin lived in the Negev. After 1948, most were expelled to Jordan and Sinai. Only around 11,000 survived in Israel (IWGIA, 2012). The position of Latin America and the Caribbean is after Africa, with about 40 million Indigenous people. The circumstances of each people are unique, but as Indigenous peoples they also face common problems and challenges.

National Household Survey (NHS) estimates that in Canada there are 1,400,685 people with an Aboriginal identity in 2011, representing 4.3 percent of the total Canadian population (Statistics Canada, 2014). The highest percentage of Aboriginal people live in Ontario and the western provinces (Manitoba, Saskatchewan, Alberta, and British Columbia) and they make up the largest shares of the population of Nunavut and the Northwest Territories. The Indigenous people in Alaska are called Alaskan Natives, who make up 16 percent of the Alaskan population of 663,661 (US Census, 2012). The small-numbered Indigenous peoples number approximately 250,000 individuals in total and thus make up less than 0.2 percent of Russia's population. They traditionally inhabit huge territories, stretching from the Kola Peninsula in the west to the Bering Strait in the east, and make up about two-thirds of the Russian territory (IWGIA, 2012).

Interestingly, Indigenous populations constitute nearly 15 percent of the total population of New Zealand. The Indigenous peoples of Australia are the Indigenous Australians, who account for 2.4 percent of the total population (2001 census figures). The independent state of Papua New Guinea (PNG) has a majority population of Indigenous societies, with some 700+ different tribal groups recognized.

Indigenous people are defined as people having historical ties to a land that outdate other people who reside there. Though, in fact, no one has lived anywhere for an unlimited amount of time, Indigenous people simply have adopted a way of life in response to the conditions that the land they come from brings. As colonizers came and settled new lands, Indigenous people were faced with a challenge in trying to readjust living in accordance with the new dynamics they were faced with. Migrating colonizers reduced the Indigenous populations by introduction of diseases, forced exploitation, war, as well as among many other push factors. For the Indigenous people who stayed in their ancestral homeland, sometimes pull factors compelled them to eventually take up and leave the land that they had historical roots in for centuries. Long after the death of the colonial age came the age of globalization, and though maybe not all the Indigenous people have experienced such an external push forcing them off their land since colonial times, the new age of globalization can bring about an internal desire as well as other external factors that change the way of life among Indigenous people.

The change brought about can be described as good or bad, but surely it is life changing. The Maasai people of Tanzania and Kenya, for example, have been able to cope with drought with the use of cell phone technology that was implemented due in part to the Kenyan government. Whether this is disrupting the traditional order that the Maasai have relied on is subject to debate; however, what is fact is that globalization means even the most remote people have access to new tools that give them ease in carrying out everyday functions. For the Maasai the cell phone can become something desired; however, as it becomes more popular it perhaps threatens the traditional way the Maasai have lived. Reading the land has been a way of life for nomadic people, and the use of technology places less reliance on the reading and more is communicated socially with the assistance of technology. Whether this is something good or not is debatable, but what holds true is that the introduction of the cell phone has changed the way of life for the Maasai people. Furthermore, Maasai people have started deepen their reliance on mobile phones in the way that they use it to communicate about market prices, and that in itself has brought them closer to the market and thus has changed their source of living (Santos, 2010).

What fed the rise of globalization was the creation of the nation-state, and because of the boundaries imposed by the nation, the people contained within those boundaries became limited to the state itself. As shown above, it depends on the perspective as to whether globalization is a hazard to the people. Another example would be the Bedouin people. For the Bedouin Arabs, the desert was an open place to move about in. Today, the Bedouins of Israel are contained not only within Israeli borders but also restricted in movement and constrained by what type of environment that they may live in. When the state of Israel was created, it sought to colonize the Negev desert; however, a large Indigenous population of people were present there. As a large majority of Arabs within Israeli boundaries, many Bedouins faced a fate of being relocated outside of the state borders; however, because of the nomadic Bedouin lifestyle of moving around constantly, the Israeli government was unable to remove the Indigenous population and in response tried to an extent to integrate the Bedouins into Israeli society (Sadik, 2013).

Though the Bedouins of Israel are Arab citizens and thus represent a minority within a minority, they have integrated to a much larger extent than other Arab citizens. They are no longer known commonly as Israeli Arabs but rather Negev Bedouins to differentiate themselves from other Bedouin Arabs in neighboring countries. Along with a name differentiation, the Negev Bedouins have changed to a large extent their cultural and traditional way of life (Sadik, 2013). They no longer are strictly nomadic because of the boundaries imposed by the Israeli government; today about more than half of the Bedouins live in the seven government-built Bedouin towns, with the remaining population residing in 46 different villages; of which only 11 are officially recognized by the state. Among the 35 unofficially recognized today, there remains an issue between the villages and the Israeli government; the Israeli government has ordered the demolition of many 'illegal' villages because it claims that the villages lack basic infrastructure such as water and plumbing and leave the residents stuck in poverty (Sadik, 2013). In response, the Israeli government has built new settlements and tried to attract the Bedouins to live there at low cost. Because the Bedouins have one of the highest growth rates in the world (more than 5 percent annually), they add to the 'Israeli demographic threat' of an overpopulating Arab majority. In theory, by educating and integrating the Bedouins into Israeli society, Israelis will not see them as a threat and they will contribute to the state. As they change their way of life, their growth rates may lessen, lowering the demographic threat Israel perceives. Overall, although states like Israel make the claim that they are seeking to improve the quality of life for people like the Bedouins by modernizing them, they in fact are also taking away the traditional way of society for them and introducing a new one. Even though it make it may increase the health of the average Bedouin and improve life expectancy and mortality rate, it can be argued that the change in lifestyle is one that forced upon them and therefore has negative conations attached to it (Sadik, 2013).

Indigenous people are scattered all over the world, and this chapter attempts to respect this fact; the vast body of literature on Indigenous population, however, has so far focused mainly on those groups residing in the high-income countries of Australia, Aoteatora/New Zealand, Canada and the USA. Indigenous peoples are spread all over Asia, Africa, the Arctic, Australia, Europe, the Pacific, North America, Central America and South America. They hold their own unique cultural names for their distinct cultural identities such as the San, the Inuit, the Ainu, the Wiradjuri, the Sami/Saami, the Maori, the Mayan, the Navajo and the Zapara (Durey and Thompson, 2012). Research conducted on these peoples bear out that by all indicators, these populations have worse health than non-Indigenous. In addition to the heath disparity, they also suffer cultural erosion. According to the United Nations (2009), of the around 7,000 languages, more than 4,000 are spoken by Indigenous peoples; however, about 90 percent of the world's languages are likely to become extinct or threatened with extinction by the end of the century—meaning that they are going to face grave danger (United Nations, 2009).

Objectives and Significance: In many countries such as Canada, Australia and New Zealand, the issue of the health of Aboriginal people has become a national priority. Studies have been done before to investigate how the burden of diseases affects Indigenous life. Identification of about 170 kinds of diseases that ravage the life of the Indigenous was made. However, not a lot of studies were conducted on what factors much matter for their health. It is a reality that priority setting is crucial to set meaningful health strategies. However, it is equally important to identify the roots of health problems of the Indigenous. To this end, a precise understanding of the Indigenous health and social determinants of health is required.

Though Indigenous health may be set as a priority, there are gaps in the state of health between Indigenous and non-Indigenous in all the countries in the world. It therefore remains a longstanding challenge for any government to improve Indigenous health. Social determinants theory contends that health and inequality is determined by many inter-linked social factors (Australian Institute of Health and Welfare and Australian Bureau of Statistics, 2005). In chapter 3, I have discussed social determinants of Indigenous health in a wide perspective. Indigenous communities lack equal access to primary health care and maintain lower standards of health infrastructure (healthy housing, food, sanitation etc.) compared to the dominant group.

Lives of the Indigenous have been ravaged by many factors, including diseases, changes in their habitat, forced displacement from their land, civil wars, and the need to adapt to drastically different habits and lifestyles. It is believed that globalization has brought Indigenous peoples powerful allies, a louder voice that can be heard internationally, and increased political influence at home (Naim, 2003). When members of the Igorot Indigenous tribe in northern Philippines and the Brunca tribe from Costa Rica gather in Geneva, their collaboration helps to extend the survival of their respective ways of life, even if they choose to compare notes over a Quarter Pounder in one of that city's many McDonalds (Naim, 2003).

The first UN publication on the state of the world's Indigenous peoples reveals alarming statistics on poverty, health, education, employment, human rights, the environment and more. Indigenous peoples all over the world continue to suffer from disproportionally high rates of poverty, health problems, crime and human rights abuses.

- In the United States, a Native American is 600 times more likely to contract tuberculosis and 62 percent more likely to commit suicide than the general population.
- In Australia, an Indigenous child can expect to die 20 years earlier than his non-native compatriot. The life expectancy gap is also 20 years in Nepal, while in Guatemala it is 13 years and in New Zealand it is 11.
- In parts of Ecuador, Indigenous people have 30 times greater risk of throat cancer than the national average.
- Worldwide, more than 50 percent of Indigenous adults suffer from Type 2 diabetes—a number predicted to rise.
- Indigenous peoples experience disproportionately high levels of maternal and infant mortality, malnutrition, cardiovascular illnesses, HIV/AIDS and other infectious diseases, such as malaria and tuberculosis.

Suicide rates of Indigenous peoples, particularly among youth, are considerably higher in many countries—for example, up to 11 times the national average for the Inuit in Canada (UN, 2010).

This book's research objective relates "globalization" to the health of Indigenous people (IP), through the analytical framework of "social determinants of health" (SDH), especially the control of the same through self-determination (self-governance, self-rule, self-control, autonomy, etc.). The UNDRIP has been cited as an exhortation to self-determination, using the modern discourse of rights, and therefore control over SDH, and therefore potential improvement in the health of IPs.

Methodological Issues: "There is no definitive Indigenous research model or methodologies. The focus is on the need for reorientation and adaption of the research business, and in its practice, of researchers' worldviews and of standard methodologies and instruments" (Putt, 2013: 2).

I wrote a report in 2007 on Indigenous population and globalization. This report basically tried to locate Indigenous populations in the domain of globalization. In doing so, I found that their status and the treatment (social and health services) they are receiving from the governments and non-Indigenous population are the consequences of colonial legacy. Ever since, we have looked for literature and available research. Over the last seven years, our quest for research on Indigenous populations and how have they been subordinated to non-Indigenous counterpart and how colonial legacy has had impact on their health, livelihood and overall liberty has ended up with some pressing issues: while there is lot of research done on Indigenous populations, only a handful of them covered social determinants of health of Indigenous peoples; a few of them covered these issues across continents, leaving the opportunity of comparing the Indigenous situations. This volume is an effort to bridge the knowledge gap that exists in the scholarship of Indigenous health. To that end, a number of researchers began to collect information from different countries (in Oceania, Latin America, North America, Europe, Africa, Asia) in the world. The research that this volume is based on applied both primary and secondary data. The secondary data used were collected through policy papers, analytical reports, various conference reports and UN systems policy papers. I selected the researchers based on their interest, logistical convenience and research experiences in relevant area. In selecting researchers, I prioritized locals and Indigenous people. I selected one Bangladeshi student who had been in Australia for about six years. One of our authors spent a substantial amount of time in Chittagong Hill Tracts, where around half a million Indigenous people live. One researcher spent about a month in India to collect data. One Finnish researcher worked for about six months in Finland and Norway and supplied qualitative data. Another researcher spent about a month in South East Asia.

The pressing issue in the course of our research was how to determine research methods given the fact that social and political settings are distinct from one country to another. The complexity of the particular research that this volume is built on took specific shapes. For instance, researchers were not from Indigenous groups that they engaged in research on. The challenges were oftentimes insurmountable. Immersion into the Indigenous community was one of the major challenges for those who were not well prepared.

A number of core values characterize good practice in social sciences, including respect for subjects or participants; voluntary participation; informed consent; and ensuring privacy and confidentiality. Researchers collected data by attending Indigenous events. A verbal consent was obtained before they were allowed to join their events. The use of narratives is a method that works well to lead researchers down many paths of knowledge creation (Weber-Pillwax, 2004). Some other methods used include informal interviews, focus groups, and sharing ideas in informal events, such as cultural programs and dances.

Most of our researchers began to initiate personal contacts through telephone calls, giving some small gifts to their children, and offering tea or coffee. A rapport building was important to gain access to these community. At a point of time, the communities began to trust them. Our researchers were sometimes even invited to family events, such as wedding ceremonies. Experiences gathered through the long time of immersion confirmed our hypothesis.

Of course, at some point, I used snowballing technique to select specific communities and their activities and events. I spent some time explaining the purpose of our visit and how this work is in the long run going to have impact on the communities. Interestingly, I and my research team were always welcomed by them. With community acceptance, conducting research may be jeopardized. I changed and improved our ways of doing research based on the mistakes made before. As mentioned, snowballing has been one of the important ways of selecting communities, and I used my own personal networks of friends as well. The influence of culture in selecting methods for particular research is always critical.

As states like Israel seek to integrate the citizens within their borders, Indigenous people are transformed in order to fit the mold of the nation-state. However, even though this is happening in the modern day, the notion of forcing the Indigenous people to conform to the state may be just as old as the nation-state itself. What is happening more today is Indigenous people transforming in the larger global context. Papua New Guinea may have a population of over 7 million; however, within these 7 million people, there are estimated to be over 800 spoken languages (Country Health Information Profiles, 2010). One aspect of globalization is the spread of a global language—which is most likely English in the contemporary sense. One of Papua New Guinea's three official languages is English, and just as in Papua New Guinea, the use of English is growing rapidly throughout the world. Once people learn English, they are more able to utilize their global citizenship and transmit ideas, especially through the use of technological instruments like the Internet. As they intermingle more with a global social network, they become more a part of it and thus leave part of their traditional society. As English use increases throughout the world, it allows the ease of spreading ideas and thus may add more to a central dominant way of thought, but at the same time it eliminates the essence of host cultures as more English/global elements are added to the host societies. Again, whether the use of English adds or subtracts from the Indigenous people's health is debatable; while it depletes the traditional way of medicine, it allows more ease of access to things like health websites that may permit people to help self-diagnose themselves.

Though the last examples included a lot of issues that are subject to debate, something factual that harms the health of Indigenous peoples is the depletion of the natural environment that they reside in. Because globalization entails the rise of the automobile and other fossil fuel burning technologies, a rise in greenhouse gas emissions has also occurred in the recent century. A surplus of greenhouse gasses has been linked with the depletion of the ozone, especially in the polar regions of the globe. For Indigenous people living there, like the Inuit of North America, the rise in greenhouse gasses has also been linked to a rise in temperature, or what has been termed as 'global warming,' and has been seen as a threat to their existence. During the week of April 20–24, 2009, a summit was held in Anchorage, Alaska, to discuss Indigenous people's right to climate change decisions made by other big organizations. The end result was what became known as the Anchorage Declaration, expressing 14 different stances that Indigenous people of the Arctic hold in response to what climate change has brought and ways they can overcome the environmental deprivation. The reliance Indigenous people of the Arctic have on the environment is the reliance most other Indigenous people have with mother earth. A statement that comes to summarize that more in depth:

> Through our knowledge, spirituality, sciences, practices, experiences and relationships with our traditional lands, territories, waters, air, forests, oceans, sea ice, other natural resources, and all life, Indigenous Peoples have a vital role in defending and healing Mother Earth. The future of Indigenous Peoples lies in the wisdom of our elders, the restoration of the sacred position of women, the youth of today and in the generations of tomorrow.
>
> (The Anchorage Declaration, 2009)

Again, as Indigenous people face destruction and transformation of their natural habitat, they, as I saw with the Negev Bedouins, are forced into assimilating into a new lifestyle; however, while the state of Israel claims it is doing it for the good of the people, it is much harder to argue that destroying the Earth's natural atmosphere does any human good. In the case of the Anchorage Declaration, Indigenous people are speaking out for their own survival, human rights and restoration of the land ("We call upon states to return and restore lands, territories, waters, forests, oceans, sea ice and sacred sites that have been taken from Indigenous Peoples, limiting our access to our traditional ways of living, thereby causing us to misuse and expose our lands to activities and conditions that contribute to climate change"). Furthermore, Indigenous people are reliant upon the land on which they live, and as this land becomes altered they are more prone to migrate. As the Anchorage Declaration goes on to claim:

> In particular, States must ensure that Indigenous Peoples have the right to mobility and are not forcibly removed or settled away from their traditional lands and territories, and that the rights of Peoples in voluntary isolation are

upheld. In the case of climate change migrants, appropriate programs and measures must address their rights, status, conditions, and vulnerabilities.

(The Anchorage Declaration, 2009)

The Anchorage Declaration is one that may have been highly influenced by the UN's Declaration on the Rights of Indigenous Peoples, which was created two years prior to the summit in Alaska. The Declaration emphasized the right of Indigenous people to maintain their traditions and societies and also prohibited discrimination against Indigenous people. However, to what extent are international rights like the UN's Declaration on the Human Rights of Indigenous Peoples respected? Australia, Canada, New Zealand and the United States, all countries with large Indigenous populations, voted against the proposition, while many countries, including Brazil, voted in favor. Marginalization or social exclusion is something the Declaration sought to fight against; however, even Brazil, a country that voted in favor of it, has some current issues with its Indigenous population (UN, 2007).

The host of the 2014 World Cup was Brazil. Where the stadium is located in Rio De Janeiro, there has been a court order to demand the exit of an Indigenous community that relocated to the area around the stadium after it was abandoned in 1977. As redevelopment occurs around the stadium, it is not clear what the Indigenous people should do, or where they should go (Watts, 2013). As globalization continues, the focus tends to be on development, and in response it usually marginalizes the native population to the corners of society. Even though Brazil was in favor of the UN's Declaration on the Human Rights of Indigenous Peoples, to express the view that the 2014 World Cup is something more important than the rights of the Indigenous people who reside within the vicinity gives the understanding that development is more important than human rights. The purpose of such organizations like the United Nations is to promote global governance and with global governance comes the rise of globalization. If development is key to globalization, then the opposite of globalization would be un-development, and since Indigenous people usually seek to maintain a traditional way of life that is untouched by economic development's expansion, then the rise of globalization may very well be the decline of Indigenous people (UN, 2007).

Just as it is with the Indigenous Brazilians, Native Alaskans, the Negev Bedouins and even the Maasai people of East Africa, the rise of globalization surely brings one thing: a change in lifestyle. Whether that is something positive or not may be debatable. Though it helps in times of drought, reshaping education systems also forces native populations to move away from a location and a traditional way of life. Health is usually measured by mortality rates, morbidity, life expectancy and many other factors. Though it may be found that in some instances these measurements start to reflect positive statistics as Indigenous people integrate into larger societies that are in the globalized loop, many other Indigenous people are left out, marginalized, and therefore at risk. So whether globalization has a positive or negative impact on health issues one can dispute; however, one thing certain is that in any case all Indigenous people who come into contact with globalization are at risk for cultural extinction.

Is it not a surprising fact that in the twenty-first century Indigenous people from the Amazon rainforest in Brazil emerge to make first-ever contact with the outside world (Gannon, 2014)? These isolated tribes have been facing severe threats of disease and violence as they have moved into new territory and encountered other people. Some people think that these people crossed into Brazil from Peru to escape drug traffickers and illegal loggers who had started working in their territory. Advocates warned this could be a deadly development. As they travel, the tribes may be at risk of contagious diseases to which they have no immunity (Gannon, 2014).

In his historic lecture on "Why Did Human History Unfold Differently on Different Continents for the Last 13,000 Years," Diamond (2001) says "it looks like a majority of his audience is of old-world origin—Eurasian or African. Yet, we could have been at this spot 500 years ago, everybody at this spot 500 years ago would have been of native American origin" (Diamond, 2001: 3–4). The peoples of Europe and eastern Asia around the globe dominate the modern world in wealth and power, while other peoples, including the original inhabitants of Australia, the Americas, and southern Africa, are no longer even masters of their own lands but have been decimated, subjugated, or exterminated by European colonialists. Why did history turn out that way, instead of the opposite way? Why weren't Native Americans, Africans, and Aboriginal Australians the ones who conquered or exterminated Europeans and Asians (Diamond, 2001)? What would happen to the history of Gypsies or today's Indigenous population if history unfolded in the reverse way? What would happen to Gypsies' (cultural) foreignness and their (social) marginality, and their rejection by the majority European populations (Smith, 2008)?

The persisting inequities the Indigenous peoples have been experiencing are irrespective of the country or region widening. In terms of health, income poverty and education, the gap between Indigenous and non-Indigenous population is well known. Health inequities are of grave concern from a public health perspective, but also from a human rights perspective (Olivera, 2012). Let us take a look at a few determinants of health (mental health, Infant and Child Mortality among Indigenous Peoples, nutrition and Communicable Diseases) of the Indigenous populations. Infant mortality rates in many regions have declined; however, for the Indigenous children in comparison to the rest of the population, they have increased. Indigenous peoples have poorer mental health outcomes and higher rates of disability due to injuries and accidents than their non-Indigenous counterparts. Diseases as well continue to disproportionately affect Indigenous peoples around the globe. Poor nutrition is one of the health issues that most affects Indigenous peoples around the world (IASG, 2014).

Chapter Organization

This book is composed of seven chapters. Chapter 1 introduces the major themes of the book, and the organization of the book's discussion is provided by this explanation of the purpose of each chapter. The second chapter deals with the conceptual account of the Indigenous peoples around the world. There are widespread misunderstandings about the definitions and locations of Indigenous populations. *Indigenous* refers to people comprising a group or culture regarded as coming from a given place; by this definition, this means almost any person or group is Indigenous to some location or other. As a contemporary cultural description, however, *Indigenous* has a much narrower meaning, describing people whose everyday lives and livelihood are governed largely by their own tradition and custom.

The following chapter (chapter 3) analyzes social determinants of health (education, employment, poverty incidents, inequality, life expectancy, social status etc.) of the Indigenous and where they figure in terms of health in global context. Many functions held by the nation-state through globalization are transferred upwards to supranational institutions and common markets through economic and political integration, downwards to regions and communities through political and administrative decentralization, and sideways to NGOs and the private sector through 'democratization' and privatization. This chapter, therefore, discusses how Indigenous populations play out in these dynamics.

Chapter 4 demonstrates the interplay of SDH and self-determination. While there is extensive diversity in Indigenous peoples throughout the world, all Indigenous Peoples have one thing in common—they all share a history of injustice and deprivation: they have been denied rights, killed, tortured and enslaved. Throughout the world, with a few exceptions, they have been suffering an overwhelming aggression against the Rights of Indigenous Peoples by colonial powers and by other nations. They continue to face threats to their very existence due to systematic exclusionary policies of their respective governments.

Chapter 5 deals with the fact that Indigenous populations struggle with the injustices regarding their displacement from the land or denial of access to the land to enjoy their own cultural mores. The colonially generated cultural disruption that affected First Nations compounds the effects of dispossession to create near total psychological, physical and financial dependency on the state. In such circumstances, opportunities for a self-sufficient, healthy and autonomous life became very limited.

Chapter 6 discusses relevant policies, governance and international processes that concern the plight of the Indigenous. As a result of the concerns of international organizations and the tireless efforts of the Indigenous, the UNHRC adopted the UN Declaration on the Rights of Indigenous Peoples (UDRIP). The last chapter (Chapter 7) summarizes the entire book and formulates some policy recommendations for the Indigenous leaders and International community.

2　Locating the Indigenous Peoples

There are widespread misunderstandings about the definitions and locations of Indigenous populations. While studies are abundant on the Indigenous populations, no clear indication or estimate are so far available about their locations. This chapter provides conceptual accounts of the Indigenous peoples around the world and attempts to analyze the existing definitions to come up with a unified and solid definition of *Indigenous*. Broadly, *Indigenous* refers to people comprising a group or culture regarded as coming from a given place; by this definition, this means almost any person or group is Indigenous to some location or other. As a contemporary cultural description, however, *Indigenous* has a much narrower meaning, describing people whose everyday lives and livelihood are governed largely by their own tradition and custom.

The most commonly used approaches to defining Indigenousness are the language spoken, self-perception and geographic concentration. Indigenous peoples are generally regarded as the descendants of the original inhabitants of areas that have become occupied by more powerful outsiders, and whose language, culture and religion remain distinct from the dominant group. They are the inheritors and practitioners of unique ways of relating to other people and to the environment, retaining social, cultural, economic and political characteristics that are distinct from those of the dominant and mainstream societies (Varennes, 2012). At the same time, they also frequently suffer both discrimination and pressure to assimilate into their mainstream societies. And while a concern common to most Indigenous people is that their cultural uniqueness is being lost, dominant understandings of Indigenousness often conflate authenticity with objectification. 'Authentic' Indigenousness thus becomes defined by objective and observable traits (i.e. clothing and behaviors) that conform to the dominant definitions of what it is to be a member of this Indigenous population (Hornborg, 1994; Callister, Didham and Kivi, 2009).

Jose R. Martinez-Cobo offered a working definition of Indigenous peoples:

> Indigenous communities, peoples and nations are those which, having a historical continuity with pre-invasion and pre-colonial societies that developed on their territories, consider themselves distinct from other sectors of the societies now prevailing on those territories, or parts of them. They form

at present non-dominant sectors of society and are determined to preserve, develop and transmit to future generations their ancestral territories, and their ethnic identity, as the basis of their continued existence as peoples, in accordance with their own cultural patterns, social institutions and legal system

(Netherlands Centre for Indigenous Peoples (NCIP), 2010)

When these traits are not portrayed, as is the case with Indigenous peoples in Paraguay, for instance, the authenticity of their claim to being Indigenous is regarded as 'inauthentic.' The same has been said of those Indigenous people who pursue economic and political goals that do not conform to dominant ideas of their Indigenousness (Blaser et al., 2008: 48). "Self-identification, which Article 1 of ILO Convention No 169 describes as a fundamental criterion for determining who may be considered Indigenous, is almost non-existent, most likely due to the complete lack of discourse on Indigenous peoples' rights in Eritrea" (ILO and ACPHR, 2009: 4).

By any reckoning, Indigenous peoples are regarded as one of the largest vulnerable segments of society. While differing significantly in terms of culture, identity, economic systems, and social institutions, Indigenous peoples as a whole most often reflect specific disadvantage in terms of social indicators, economic status, and quality of life.

Demographics of the Indigenous

Broadly, 'Indigenous' refers to people comprising a group or culture regarded as coming from a given place, meaning that any person or group is Indigenous to some location or other (World Bank, 1993; Reading, 2002). No single definition can identify an Indigenous population. However, there are understandings based on many factors that indicate whether a population can be considered Indigenous (UNPFII Factsheet, 2010).

Despite their cultural differences, Indigenous peoples around the world share common problems related to the protection of the rights (Raphael, 2001) to their lands, natural resources and culture. They have been seeking recognition of their identities, their ways of life, and territories and natural resources for a long time. Their voices have remained unheard by colonialists. In recent times, it seems policy makers, respective governments and the United Nations have begun to listen to their plights. The globalization of communication in recent decades is playing a positive role in this respect. Yet they remain among the most disadvantaged and vulnerable groups across the world.

With varying sizes across the world, Indigenous peoples represent approximately 5 percent of the population of the world. However, they constitute about 15 percent of the world's poor, living in more than 70 countries. About 70 percent of them live in Asia. They make up about one-third of the world's extremely poor rural people (Hall and Patrinos, 2010; IFAD, 2010; Indigenous World, 2013). In China, ethnic minority groups make up less than 9 percent of total population (World Bank, 2013). In 2001, about 90 percent of Australia's Indigenous population were identified as being of Aboriginal origin, 6 percent as being of Torres Strait Islander origin and 4 percent as being of both Aboriginal and Torres Strait Islander origin (Australian Bureau of Statistics, 2010). While in general it has been ingrained in our mind that Indigenous peoples are the minority group, there are some countries where they are not a minority; for instance, they make up more than half the population in Bolivia and Guatemala (UNDP, 2010).

Indigenous people often have unique practices that help identify and differentiate their populations from those among which they live. These characteristics include everything from cultural practices to social, political, and economic ways of life (UNPFII Factsheet, 2010). In the modern context, Indigenous populations have been pushed to submissive places in many aspects of society. At many different times in history and in many diverse global regions, this has occurred through conquest, occupation, colonization, settlement and displacement. It is essential to recognize that Indigenous populations are inherently separate from those in which they currently live. They exist in a distinct fashion, where self-recognition and identification are essential, but simultaneously they live within a society that dominates their way of life. The implications of living such a life are many, most notably in health access and employment.

People in general can trace their genetic lineage and heritage to Indigenous persons, but the self-identification and existence as a population, as a self-aware and separate group, creates a more definable and distinct group. This is reinforced and further contrasted when it occurs against a backdrop of a larger, more dominant entity, such as a nation, a state, or another Indigenous group. Common ancestral links exist in many Indigenous populations, which usually span across long periods of time and last through colonization and settlement (UNPFII, 2010). The links can, and often do, include a genetic heritage, but also can be attached to territories, regions, resources, and other means of identification. In the political context, since the beginning of the nineteenth century, some levels of protection have been extended to Indigenous people through international treaties (Lile, 2006: 9). However, globalization and the rise in international focus have left Indigenous peoples under the purview of domestic authorities. This shift has resulted in Indigenous populations becoming marginalized and, in some cases, oppressed.

Several studies have confirmed that there is a correlation between being Indigenous and high incidences of poverty, with very little or no improvement as time passes (Hall and Patrinos, 2006: 2). This includes a disconnect between Indigenous populations and socioeconomic access. Irrespective of countries, developed or developing, Indigenous populations have far lower rates of access to education, jobs, health services, and local economies.

The formation of the United Nations Permanent Forum on Indigenous Issues (UNPFII) marked the first major step of advocacy for Indigenous peoples from outside the domestic arena.

> If there is one thing that all Indigenous peoples in the world have in common it is that they have been oppressed by their own government and they do not want the government to speak on their behalf. International institutions that

can voice the Indigenous peoples own concerns and provide pressure on the governments is essential for Indigenous peoples.

(Lile, 2006: 1)

However, the growth in national and international political priorities has contin-ued and still continues to sideline major issues of inequality for Indigenous popu-lations. In the 1990s and 2000s, several uprisings occurred across Latin America as a result of increasingly marginalized treatment.

Hall and Patrinos (2006: 1) said:

> The year 1994 heralded a major uprising of Indigenous people in the Mexi-can state of Chiapas, known as the Zapatista rebellion. Deploring the world's lack of attention to their plight, the actions of these people signaled the begin-ning of a new era in which Indigenous peoples would play an increasingly vocal part in national politics.

The results of these movements have been mixed, but changes in domestic leg-islation, constitutional protection, and even entire regime changes have occurred because of pushes for Indigenous rights, particularly in Latin America. Addition-ally, international development organizations, such as the ILO and the World Bank, among others, have also adopted similar changes in their policies when dealing with countries that have Indigenous populations, with an aim for greater protection.

Hall and Patrinos (2006) aimed to look at development markers to see if the previously mentioned changes expanded the rights and access of Indigenous populations to a variety of socioeconomic factors. The idea of markers is to see if the previously mentioned changes expanded the rights and access of Indig-enous populations to a variety of factors such as economy, opportunities and culture. The goal is to identify markers that would help make policy recom-mendations on a global and international understanding of poverty. In the late 1990s and early 2000s, political representation of Indigenous populations saw a rise. There is evidence that there is an enhanced participation in representa-tion in policy-making levels, even in high-level offices such as presidencies, mayorships, vice-presidencies and members of parliaments (Hall and Patrinos, 2006: 3).

Locating the Indigenous

According to the discussion above on the definition, Indigenous people can be found in most of the regions in the world. Here, we are presenting the popula-tion with regional data, which is most important for readers to analyze to better understand the dynamics of Indigenous populations in terms of their sizes, histori-cal deprivations, longstanding struggles for equal rights, and policies that are in place. We attempt to locate Indigenous peoples in the Indigenous Global Coordi-nating Group (GCG) regions. The GCG is composed of seven Indigenous regions.

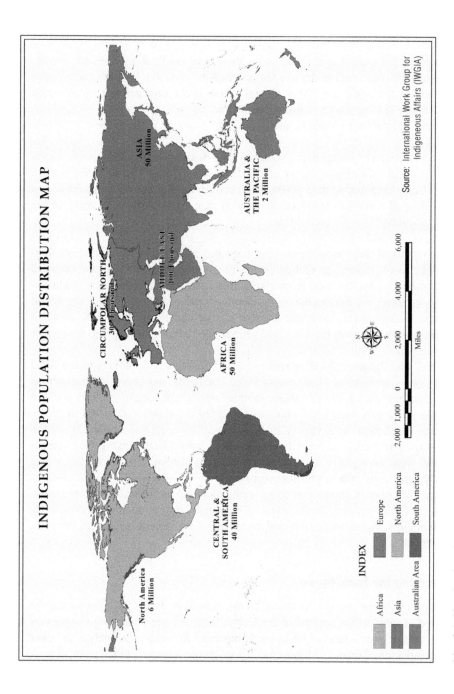

Map 2.1 Showing locations and number of Indigenous populations

African and Middle Eastern Region

There are about 50 million Indigenous people in Africa. In this region, Indigenous peoples face the highest number of challenges, ranging from marginalization and non-recognition by governments and other ethnic groups, to poverty, AIDS/HIV, and illiteracy (Sakuda, 2004). They have been nomadic and seminomadic pastoralists and hunters. Despite a general trend towards state assimilation, Indigenous

Table 2.1 Indigenous populations in the Middle East and Africa

Countries	Number of Indigenous people	% of total population
Middle East Region		
Israel	53,111 + 148,729 Bedouin	
Palestine	3.9 Million	
North and West African Region		
Morocco	9 Million (the number of Amazigh speakers)	28
Algeria	11 Million (Tamazight speakers)	33
Mali	1.5 million	10
Niger	1,248,914 Peul + 1,219,528 Tuareg + 220,397 Toubou = 2.6 Million	17
Burkina Faso	(not known)	
East African Region		
Kenya	25% of the national population	
Uganda	260,117+	
Tanzania	Maasai in Tanzania at 430,000; the Datoga group to which the Barabaig belongs at 87,978; the Hadzabe at 1,000 and the Akie (Ndorobo is derogatory) at 5,268	
Central African Region		
Burundi	78,071	1
Democratic Republic of Congo (DRC)	About 600,000 Pygmies (while civil society organizations argue that there are up to 2,000,000 (3% of the population)	1
Cameroon	68,000 (Pygmies)	0.4
Central African Republic	Mbororo population of 39,299	1
Southern African Region		
Namibia	27,000–34,000 The San (Bushmen)	1.5
Botswana	68,000	3.4
Zimbabwe	14,000	.1
South Africa	500,000	1

Source: The Indigenous World (2013).

peoples' organizations in Africa are mobilizing to make their voices heard and advocate their cause (IWGIA, 2013).

In countries where Indigenous populations form the basis for a considerable portion of the population, lower than proportional voter turnout and representation was still seen among them. Even as this has occurred, a rise in Indigenous-influenced NGOs has corresponded to increased proliferation of mass movements and policy changes across many nations in the world.

In Eritrea, nationalism and other societal factors contribute to a difficult environment for Indigenous populations beginning with this idea of self-identification. The various ethnic groups, while all separate and distinct, also share many unifying characteristics in terms of lifestyle. Particularly with economic and agrarian systems, for example, the different ethnic groups in Eritrea, while maintaining distinct characteristics, are often forced to interact and prioritize on an economic subsistence level, which inevitably leads to less focus on individual sustainability and distinction of each of the groups themselves (ILO and ACPHR, 2008: 4).

The wars between Eritrea and Ethiopia (the Eritrean War of Independence and the later border conflict between Eritrea and Ethiopia, which resulted in the UNMEE peacekeeping mission to patrol disputed territories) contributed to the need for and the growth of Eritrean nationalism over the past 60 years. Eritrea, as a much smaller nation (which was viewed by Ethiopia as a separatist movement), now relies on a strongly enforced sense of nationalism with the goals of maintaining identity and security.

One of the means through which this is propagated is the use of compulsory national military service. In the "modern sense, regardless of ethnic groups, mandatory conscription inherently supports an idea of nationalism as paramount to any other distinct groups" (UNHCR, 2011).[1]

Self-identification is widely agreed to as a necessary marker for the legitimacy of an Indigenous population. For many ethnic groups in Eritrea, in particular, this has become incredibly difficult to see as the discourse on Indigenous issues has yet to fully 'infiltrate' in the would-be Indigenous populations.

In Eritrea, for instance, there are no official policies in place that are meant to reduce the stigmatization and marginalization of certain ethnic groups. But there are some other markers that promote stigmatization and marginalization of certain ethnic groups, especially minority groups.

Ethnic groups that have traditionally been associated with certain territories and natural resources have come under scrutiny and been the target of derogatory discrimination and marginalization because they have been less than apt to merge with modern Eritrea. Other ethnic groups are more flexible toward contemporary changes. These groups have often marginalized the more traditional groups, often by incorporating elements of racism and discrimination based on skin color.

In addition to political nationalism threatening the ways of life of Indigenous people, other political changes that are less overt also have forced Indigenous populations to adapt. Specific policies, for example, have been employed by the government in Eritrea to promote the deterioration of Indigenous identity. Pastoralism, for instance, has been threatened by specific policies of the government to encourage people to move into villages. With settling has also come further efforts by the government to incentivize integration, such as using the vaccination of cattle as a method of pushing Indigenous people to rely on government resources and external help.

The historical development of Africa is also significant for several reasons. The multiple colonial powers that at several points ruled Africa left lasting legacies of marginalization of Indigenous populations. Social divisions continued well through colonization and subsequent border disputes. The implementation of political boundaries and regional structures, for example, has incorporated Indigenous populations into the political structure of the nation but simultaneously has reinforced centralization of power and the co-opting of all Indigenous cries for independence into the national narrative of Eritrean patriotism (ILO, 2008: 17).

> The government, at least in its rhetoric, is against any form of discrimination (particularly ethnically-based) and it also sharply denies any allegation that any ethnic group is facing marginalization and discrimination. Nevertheless, since the days of the independence struggle, a tendency towards cultural and ethnic assimilation has taken root.
>
> (ILO, 2008: 17)

The undermining of Indigenous issues has been systematically implemented and occurs alongside the undermining of ethnic issues as well. In many countries in Africa, the Indigenous populations, because of political marginalization, began to form factions among other, particularly pastoral, groups during their volatile history, which ironically increased the level of marginalization they faced because they were increasingly seen as counter to the goals of the nation. Additional proclamations and deliberate government policies have also limited ethnic involvement (and thus the involvement of Indigenous populations) in the political process. Rules and structures for government involvement do not allow populations from regions that are predominant with a single ethnicity to participate in an effective manner. The Indigenous populations of the Kunama, Nara, and Tekurir, specifically, are cited as examples of where being from one major region becomes a disadvantaged one.

In the case of Eritrea, this deliberate effort by the government to structure political power in a closed manner directly clashes with the very identifying aspects of what makes a population Indigenous. For example, the idea of having a pastoral or traditional homeland or territory is a major marker for an Indigenous population and is essential for its ability to self-identify, which also serves as another key element. When political power is purposefully structured to undermine ethnic territory, as is the case in Eritrea, it does so in a way that inherently attacks Indigenous identity.

The political structures that undermine Indigenous rights and identity inherently block any available means through which the structure can be corrected. If Indigenous people are actively dissuaded from being involved in national politics, marginalization can transform into discontent, indifference, and a major lack in political efficacy, marking a transition from detachment to resentment. One of the major drawbacks to the current situation in Eritrea is the inaction of the government in implementing and ratifying the draft constitution that was meant to be ratified after the end of a transitional period of government. The current powers have simply not ratified the document that would, theoretically, provide better protection for and legal mechanisms for the participation of Indigenous populations. The lack of implementation of the constitution renders many of the included protections toothless.

Even in cases where a deliberate effort has not been made, the inherent fabric of Indigenous identities has been threatened by government policies. In the case of Eritrea and Ethiopia, the policies of centralization and the geographic division of administration zones, particularly on the village level, have marginalized Indigenous populations. Nomadic and pastoral populations of Indigenous people are hurt by the government policies that give land rights through the regional authority of a local village. Without even going beyond the surface, the concept of enforcing land rights for nomadic populations through a centralized, stationary authority, in the form of a village, is counter-intuitive.

The incorporation of Indigenous populations into contemporary geopolitics also blurs the previously mentioned definitions of Indigenous as existing as minorities in larger groups of people. According to Hall and Patrinos (2010), for example, large populations of native Americans and aborigines now live in cities, even while maintaining a cultural association with the frontier. Their argument is that only in very rare and exceptional circumstances do completely isolated Indigenous populations exist in the world.

With this realization, the most important step to take is to identify Indigenous populations that exist within the modern backdrop of international geopolitics. Nations, cities, regions, villages, and the networks that tie them all together all force a type of participation that can, in many cases, be directly contradictory to the nature of Indigenous life.

Even among the varying definitions of what constitutes an Indigenous population, there is widespread agreement that Indigenous ways of life have come under threat. Only 600 of the 6,000 languages in the world are Indigenous languages (Crystal, 2000). However, about 2500 languages in the world are in endangerment at different levels: vulnerable; definitely endangered; severely endangered; critically endangered and extinct. Most endangered languages are tied to Indigenous identities (UNESCO, 2012). Indigenous living on the border areas of states has provided some type of insulation from central authorities. However, some government efforts have increasingly targeted border areas, for example, Tibet, India, Burma, Laos, and Vietnam (Hall and Patrinos, 2012).

What is problematic is the potential conflict that exists between states and how this has provided some type of insulation indicators that are biased toward government policies, for example, the issue of education and the permeation of language. Due to over emphasis of national language, and international languages like English, many of the traditional and indigenous languages have eroded.

The clear effort by the Ethiopian government, for example, to assimilate minorities and Indigenous people through public policy is a deliberate effort to undermine Oromo identity (Human Rights Watch, 2005). Some smaller minority communities were considered to be on the verge of disappearing completely, due to factors that include resettlement, displacement, conflict, assimilation, cultural dilution, environmental factors and loss of land (Minority Rights Group International, 2008).

Minority issues are all in some way dependent upon participation within public systems. Kurds in Iraq, Iran, Turkey and Syria are examples of some smaller minority communities. In Turkey, the 1928 switch from an Arabic-based alphabet to a Latin-based alphabet imposed on the Kurdish language was a top-down change that deliberately confronted longstanding tradition and ethnic identity (Zürcher, 2004).

Using education as a means to dilute the identity of an Indigenous population is not an effort that has been isolated to the Oromo in Ethiopia or to the Kurds in the Middle East. The methods have existed since ancient history. Yet, as global politics incorporate more efforts of "development," some cases have invariably included a more subtle approach of this theory. Hall and Patrinos go on to say that the Indigenous populations are legitimate only if they retain their cultural practices and distinction from mainstream society and politics (Hall and Patrinos, 2012). Taken in light of efforts to undermine this identity, it is not difficult to see how political efforts of "development" have undermined the very legitimacy demanded of Indigenous people by public perception.

There are many cases of Oromo people whose credibility is questioned because they lack any knowledge of Oromo culture or language, yet they retain their ethnic identity. In the case of Ethiopia, deliberate efforts by the government to phase out Oromo language, especially through teaching only in Amharic, have resulted in entire generations of people whose cultural identity is founded in political, nationalist narratives that differ from their ethnic heritage (Jackery, 2014: personal communication). One of the questions this raises, in line with the previous question, is the legitimacy of an ethnic or Indigenous identity. As languages, cultures, practices, traditional lands, and rights become undermined, and in some cases pushed toward extinction, do Indigenous identities become less legitimate?

Counter-efforts, like those of the UN Permanent Forum on Indigenous Issues, highlight the need for preservation and protective efforts of identities that have been eroded. The foundation and growth of institutions and research related to Indigenous issues has also been highlighted, as has the need for clearer definitions and understandings of Indigenous identity (Lile, 2006). A large-scale shift occurred in the trend of identifying Indigenous between government censuses and self-identification over a 30-year period. This signified a change in trends to include the self-identification of Indigenous persons with their ethnic or Indigenous backgrounds (Hall and Patrinos, 2006).

Self-identification has become essential factor with a view to achieving self-determination. The inability of public institutions to protect Indigenous rights starts with the idea that there is no single objective definition of Indigenous populations, leaving identification in an ambiguous state. As Lile (2006) points out, the ILO, which primarily served as a backbone to the more recent UNPFII, did not even establish a set definition of who fits the category of Indigenous. The ILO (which primarily served as a backbone to the mo 169) did not establish exactly who it protected, citing self-identification as paramount (ILO, 1989). However, while this is seemingly in line with protecting the self-identification of Indigenous people as a fundamental part of the identity of being Indigenous, it nevertheless exposes a major shortcoming in the legal protection schemes of Indigenous peoples as they exist in a political world.

According to the ILO's own description of Convention No 169:

> The Convention does not define who are Indigenous and tribal peoples. It takes a practical approach and only provides criteria for describing the peoples it aims to protect. Self-identification is considered as a fundamental criterion for the identification of Indigenous and tribal peoples.

The same description goes further to highlight that only 20 countries have currently ratified this convention, rendering both its definitive framework and its practical implementation largely ineffective.

Contrasting this with other international legal protections, the lack of priority that was given to the issue at the time is evident. Refugee law, for example, was created out of the perceived need for a special category of vulnerable people. The response was a wide range of international legal instruments, including the relatively immediate adoption of the 1951 Refugee Convention shortly after the formation of the UN itself (Ullah, 2014), an entire agency and oversight board, and country offices that operate worldwide with staggering budgets. Yet, despite Indigenous populations outnumbering the combined populations of refugees, internally displaced, and stateless by ten times over (UNHRC, 2015), Indigenous issues did not receive a permanent agency and voice until nearly a half century later with the formation of the UNPFII on 28 July 2000 (Lile, 2006). Further, it was not until 13 September 2007 that the UN adopted its Declaration on the Rights of Indigenous Peoples (UN, 2008). Even this, however, does not carry the weight of international law and is in the form of a declaration that is used to convey support and commitment, not as an instrument that can be enforced in and of itself. It also suffered heavy criticism for not having a clear-cut definition of the term *Indigenous*.

The Arctic

Table 2.2 Indigenous populations in the Arctic

Countries	Number of Indigenous people	% of total population
Arctic Region		
Greenland	50,000	88
Russia	250,000	0.2%
Inuit Regions of Canada	55,000	4.3% of Aboriginal population in Canada

The Americas

The size of Indigenous population of North America was unknown at the time of European colonization. The pre-Contact population of Canada and the US ranges from 900,000 to 18 million (Snipp, 1989), while it was from 4.5 to 25 million for Mexico (Alba, 1977).

In the three nations of North America—Canada, the United States and Mexico—ethnicity has varying connotations. In contemporary Mexico, the primary ethnic distinction is between the Indigenous and non-Indigenous populations. The peopling of North America has been shaped by the presence of Indigenous Americans, European colonization, African slavery, and voluntary immigration, and for Mexico, by considerable emigration. During the first 50 years, the Aboriginal population grew only 29 percent, whereas the total population far more than doubled (161 percent). This slow growth rate among the Aboriginal population occurred because of high mortality rates.

Although 200,000 Native people were estimated to inhabit Canada when the French began settlement in the early seventeenth century, less than 100,000 remained by 1867 (Anderson and Frideres, 1981). In 1548, 6 million Indigenous people were estimated to inhabit Mexico, but by 1605, only 1 million remained. At the beginning of the nineteenth century, when the colonial period came to a close, Mexico's total population stood at 6 million, roughly equivalent to the Indigenous population prior to colonization. Mexico's Indigenous population rebounded following a decline between 1900 and 1920 (Alba, 1977). Currently, there are approximately 42 million Indigenous people living in the Americas (WHO, 2006). According to the 2001 Canadian census, there are over 900,000 Aboriginal people in Canada, 3.3 percent of the country's total population.

The Indigenous peoples of Canada are collectively referred to as "Aboriginal peoples." The Constitution Act, 1982 of Canada recognizes three groups of Aboriginal peoples: Indians, Inuit and Métis. According to the 2006 census, Aboriginal peoples in Canada total 1,172,790, 3.6 percent of the population of Canada. First Nations (referred to as "Indians" in the Constitution and generally registered under Canada's Indian Act) are a diverse group of 698,025 people, representing more than 52 nations and more than 60 languages. Around 55 percent live on-reserve and 45 percent reside off-reserve in urban, rural, special access and remote areas.

The Métis constitute a distinct Aboriginal nation, numbering 389,780 in 2006, many of whom live in urban centers, mostly in western Canada. The Métis people emerged out of the relations of Indian women and European men prior to Canada's crystallization as a nation. The Inuit number 55,000 people, or 4.3 percent of the Aboriginal population. They live in 53 Arctic communities in four Land Claims regions: Nunatsiavut (Labrador); Nunavik (Quebec); Nunavut; and the Inuvialuit Settlement Region of the Northwest Territories (IWGIA, 2014).

Two-thirds of urban Aboriginal people live in western Canada, and four of the five cities with the highest proportions of Aboriginal people are in the West (Hanselmann, 2001). However, public policy discussions about Indigenous people

Table 2.3 North American Region

Countries	Number of Indigenous people	% of total population
North American Region		
Canada	1,172,790	3.6
United States of America	5.2 Million	1.7
Mexico and Central America		
Mexico	15,703,474	14
Guatemala	6,000,000	60
Nicaragua	1,444,000	20
Costa Rica	104,143	2.42

Sources: CELADE (1992); The Indigenous World (2013); various sources cited in Gnerre (1990); Healthinfonet (2000); World Bank (2000) and IWGIA (2014).

tend to focus on the reserve-based population (Foliaki et al., 2003). This includes approximately 600,000 people of First Nations descent, 290,000 Métis and 45,000 Inuit (Statistics Canada, 2001a).

The estimated 33 to 40 million Indigenous peoples in Latin America and the Caribbean alone have approximately 400 different Indigenous groups in the region with different languages, social organizations, and economies (Ling and Raphael, 2004). An overwhelming majority (90 percent) of them are sedentary subsistence farmers, descendants of the pre-Columbian Inca, Maya and Aztec peoples who live in the arid mountainous regions of the Andes and Central America. Fewer than 10 percent live in dry forests or the remote tropical rain-forests of the Amazon and Orinoco basins and Central America. Five countries (Peru, Mexico, Guatemala, Bolivia and Ecuador) account for almost 90 percent of Indigenous people in the region, with Peru and Mexico having the largest populations (Auger et al., 2004).

Interestingly, the majority of the population (around 57 percent) of some countries is constituted by the Indigenous. In Bolivia, for example, more than half of the total population is Indigenous (Table 2.4). Most of the Indigenous peoples in Bolivia are Quechua and Aymara descendants and live in the rural regions. The rest belong to different tribes and reside in the jungles and low-lands and have chosen not to be incorporated into the rest of the country's life (Klein, 1982).

Indigenous peoples in the Sierra Nevada de Santa Marta and Perijá Sierra are an important part of the 85 different ethnic groups existing in Colombia. Some 60 percent of Bolivians are Indigenous belonging to the Aymara, Chiq-uitano, Guaraní, Guarayo, Moxeno, Quechua and other smaller ethnic groups. Indigenous peoples are generally divided between the lowland or 'Indigenous' (Amazon, Chaco, and the East) and highland or 'of origin' (Andean) inhabitants (Gaviria and Raphael 2001).

Table 2.4 South American Region

Countries	Number of Indigenous people	% of total population
South American Region		
Colombia	1,450,000	3.5
Venezuela	725,128	2.7
Suriname	18,200	3.7
Ecuador	1,100,000	7.1
Peru	8 million identify themselves as Quechua	40
Bolivia	6,507,696	62
Brazil	817,000	0.42
Paraguay	108,803	2
Argentina	600,329	1.51
Chile	1,369,563	8
Belize	27,000	14.7
Panama	99,000	4.1
Honduras	110,000	2.1
El Salvador	1,000	0.02

Sources: CELADE (1992); various sources cited in Gnerre (1990) and The Indigenous World (2013).

The Pacific Region

Human occupation of Australia probably began between 50,000 and 60,000 years ago. Evidence suggests that the people who became the Aborigines came from southeastern Asia, probably by raft or canoe.[2] Whether they arrived over a relatively short period of time or over thousands of years is still uncertain (Brown, 2001). Hundreds of culturally distinct Aboriginal groups were spread across the Australian continent. They occupied a wide range of environments, from the savanna woodlands of the north to the harsh desert outback and temperate woodlands of the south. Aboriginal people traditionally lived as hunter-gatherers in small family groups, hunting, fishing, and collecting a variety of plant foods. Most groups were nomadic or seminomadic and built simple brush or bark shelters (Tebtebba, 2004).

In 2005, there were around 490,000 Indigenous people in Australia, of whom around 440,000 were Aboriginal people, 30,000 Torres Strait Islanders, and 20,000 people of both Aboriginal and Torres Strait Islander descent. Indigenous people comprise around 2.4 percent of the total Australian population (Alan et al., 2011).[3] The majority live in southeastern Australia, although northern Australia has a high proportion of Indigenous people (Riley, 2000). The largest concentrations of Indigenous populations today are in cities—often suburbs of low socioeconomic status, such as Sydney's Redfern and Mount Druitt. The state with the highest Indigenous population is New South Wales (68,941 Aborigines and Torres Strait Islanders, or 1.2 percent of the total). Next is Queensland (67,012 or

Table 2.5 The Pacific Region

Countries	Number of Indigenous people	% of total population
The Pacific Region		
Australia	520,000	2.5
Aotearoa (New Zealand)	731,000	17
Tuvalu	Total population 11,000	
New Caledonia	98,232	40
Papua New Guinea	231,835	4

Sources: Healthinfonet (2000); World Bank (2000); Statistics Canada (2005); The Indigenous World (2013) and IWGIA (2014).

2.25 percent); Western Australia (40,002 or 2.52 percent); Northern Territory (38,337 or 21.88 percent); Victoria (16,570 or 0.39 percent); South Australia (16,020 or 1.14 percent); Tasmania (8,683 or 1.92 percent); and Australian Capital Territory (1,768 or 0.63 percent) (United Nations, 2006).

New Zealand (Aotearoa) is historically a bicultural country made up basically of two ethnic components, the Maori, who trace their ancestry to the original Polynesian inhabitants, and the descendants of the European colonists and settlers, known as Pakeha, who arrived in increasing numbers beginning in the nineteenth century. New Zealand is becoming a more multicultural society because of recent immigration from the Pacific Islands, Asia, Eastern Europe and Africa. Out of a total population of about four million, the Maori, whose numbers dropped precipitously due to contact with Europeans, currently represent around 15 percent, most of whom currently live in urban centers (United Nations, 2006). Approximately 15 percent of the population claimed at least one ancestor from the country's Indigenous Maori or Moriori minorities (Tebtebba, 2004).

Papua New Guinea, the world's second largest island, became separated from the Australian mainland when the area was known as the Torres Strait flooded around 5000 BC (Tebtebba, 2004). The current population of the island of New Guinea is about 6.9 million people. The great variety of the island's Indigenous populations is frequently assigned to one of two main ethnological divisions, based on archaeological, linguistic and genetic evidence: the Papuan and Austronesian groups. The island is presently populated by very nearly a thousand different tribal groups and a near-equivalent number of separate language, all falling into one of two groups, the Papuan language and the Austronesian language. Indigenous peoples constitute four percent of the total population of Papua New Guinea (Tebtebba, 2004).

Asian Region

In Asia, there are about 200 million Indigenous people, and around half of them live in India, where 12 percent of the total population (around 100 million people) is Indigenous, living in 461 tribal communities concentrated in the central provinces of India, the middle belt and the northeastern states. About 92 percent of the tribal people in India live in rural areas (Government of India, 2010, 1991). Most of them live in areas which are either dry, forested or hilly (Shah et al., 2003). They depend on agriculture and minor forest produce for their livelihood (Patwardhan, 2007). Compared with India, China has fewer numbers of Indigenous peoples, with an estimate of 67 million (Welker, 2007). The number of Indigenous people in Thailand is between 1 million and 1.5 million. About 50 percent of the population is tribals and mainly followers of Theravada Buddhism. The highest percentage of Indigenous population in Asia (compared to the general population) lives in Nepal (36 percent) (Table 2.6).

Bangladesh's Indigenous population numbered around 900,000 in 1981, or around one percent of the total population. They live in 45 minority communities (Oxfam, 2006), primarily in the hilly areas in Bangladesh, such as Chittagong Hills and in the regions of Mymensingh, Sylhet and Rajshahi. The majority of the tribal population (almost 800,000) live in rural settings where environmental crisis is more severely felt. In Bangladesh's Indigenous territories, the agricultural frontier and the exploitation of natural resources have been destroying the habitat. Around 45 percent of the inhabitants are Bengali Muslim settlers. The remainder is followers of Hinduism, Christianity and Animism. The local tribes, collectively known as the Jumma, include the Chakma, Marma, Tripura, Tenchungya, Chak, Pankho, Mru, Murung, Bawm, Lushai, Khyang and Khumi (Ramasubramanian, 2005).

Table 2.6 South Asian Region

Countries	Number of Indigenous people	% of total population
South Asian Region		
Bangladesh	3,000,000	1.93
Nepal	9,485,032 (Adivasi Janajati) of Nepal	36
India	84.3 million	8.2
Pakistan	2,200,000	0.17
Nagalim	Approximately 4 million in population	
East and South East Asia Region		
Japan	30,782	.02
China	113,792,211	8.49
Taiwan	526,148	2.25
The Philippines	13,800,000	10–20
Indonesia	50–70 million	24
Malaysia	3,480,000	12
Thailand	923,257	1.4
Vietnam	13 million	14
Laos	one-third of 7 million	32
Burma	28 million (although the government does not recognize the existence of Indigenous peoples)	68
Cambodia	100,000	1

Sources: Healthinfonet (2000); World Bank (2000); The Indigenous World (2013) and IWGIA (2014).

As in other parts of the world, Indigenous peoples in Bangladesh are the most disadvantaged, neglected and vulnerable people in the country. The government of Bangladesh does not have any formal policy for the development of Indigenous populations. Indigenous peoples have often faced eviction from their homelands in the name of development projects and conservation such as dams, eco-parks, protected areas, reserve forests and even the establishment of military bases on their ancestral and community land. Their land has been taken without their consent. Their culture is treated as inferior in the country.

Over the years, Indigenous peoples have experienced a strong sense of social, political and economic exclusion, lack of recognition, fear and insecurity, loss of cultural identity, and social oppression. Mainstream development efforts have either ignored their concerns and/or had a negative impact on them. Often issues and actions that affect them are not discussed with these communities or organizations representing them. Thus they are subjected to stark socioeconomic deprivation. Mass relocation of non-Indigenous people in the traditional adivasi/ethnic minority areas have also caused land-grabbing, leading to livelihood displacement among the Indigenous peoples. More than 45 Indigenous ethnic communities with a population of nearly three million people have been living in the country for centuries. According to the 2001 (provisional) Census Report, the total number of Indigenous (officially 'tribal') people in Bangladesh is about 1,772,788, which is 1.28 percent of the total population of the country. However, Indigenous peoples claim that the population of the Indigenous peoples all over the country is about 3 million (AIPP, 2007).

Indigenous peoples in other parts of 'plains' Bangladesh are located mainly in the border regions in the northwest (Rajshahi-Dinajpur), central north (Mymensingh-Tangail), northeast (Greater Sylhet), south and southeast (Chittagong, Cox's Bazar and Greater Barisal). According to the 2001 (provisional) census report, the Indigenous peoples of the plain regions were estimated to number about 1,036,060. However, plain Indigenous peoples claim that their population is estimated at 2 million. Among them, the Santal are the most numerous, constituting almost 30 percent of the Indigenous population of the plains, followed by the Garo, Hajong, Koch, Manipuri, Khasi, Rakhain etc. (AIPP, 2007).

Historically, the Indigenous Jumma peoples are known to have lived in the CHT even before the arrival of the Portuguese in Bengal in the sixteenth century. On the other hand, Bengali people, who are the most populous and dominant ethnic group in Bangladesh, are not known to have settled in the region prior to the nineteenth century. However, the Bengali population has increased many times since then, especially with the government-sponsored population transfer program of 1979. According to the respondents, the more than 400,000 Bengali Muslims from the plains districts have illegally been given settlement in CHT by the government.

Europe

While Saami peoples were found well documented, literature or any study on European Indigenous is scant. Available data show that the Saami settlement area extends into four countries: Finland, Norway, Russia and Sweden. They inhabited these areas long before the establishment of state boundaries and they are therefore recognized as an Indigenous people in Norway (Tebtebba, 2004). No precise numbers are available regarding the size of the Saami population in Norway; however, estimates place it somewhere between 60,000 and 100,000. Around 15–25,000 Saami people live in Sweden, while there are over 6,000 in Finland and 2,000 in Russia. The Saami reindeer husbandry area encompasses Norway's five most northerly counties and the municipality of Engerdal in Hedmark County (Sheridan, 2001).

Roma in Europe: The inclusion of the Roma people in Central and Eastern Europe has been an issue of growing importance as a number of countries from the former Soviet Union bloc have sought entry into the European Union. One the one hand, the challenges facing the Roma minority are one of overcoming poverty, gaining access to education, and developing marketable skills (UNDP, 2002: 1); while on the other hand, reports of pervasive human rights violations of the Roma in such countries as Romania, Hungary, and others has raised concerns about the changes needed within those countries to better align with European standards on human rights. As Isabel Fonesca asserts, "the most dramatic change for Central and Eastern Europe Gypsies since the revolutions of 1989 has been the sharp escalation of hatred and violence directed toward them" (1995: 140). It had been widely recognized for years that the Roma, often referred to in a more derogatory sense as the Gypsies, have occupied a place of marginalization and social exclusion in their respective countries, yet it was the dramatic increase of human rights violations in the 1990s that finally prompted international organizations and national governments to take action. On 2 February 2005, nine Central and Eastern European countries considered to have the most significant Roma populations in the region launched the initiative The Decade of Roma Inclusion 2005–2015, committing their governments to bring about changes that would not only benefit the Roma, but the majority populations as well. In this section, I will examine some of the factors that have resulted in the Roma leading such marginalized and impoverished lives, and will look at what is being proposed to address the problem. More specifically, I will look at the Roma living in Romania and will argue that their past, which has been largely overshadowed by centuries of slavery, persecution, and social exclusion, coupled with their traditional values and earlier nomadic ways, have all contributed to the their current existence on the fringes of twenty-first century Romanian society.

Who are Gypsies? A starting point for understanding the current predicament of modern-day Gypsies is to take a look at who they are as a people, and how they came to be more recently known as the Roma. Historically, Gypsies were largely a nomadic people travelling in caravans of single or multiple families, and they lived in rural encampments on the outskirts of urban or rural areas, working in the informal sector and doing menial work (Sanborne, 1996: 104). The many tribes which make up the diverse Gypsy communities have traditionally been grouped according to their specific trades, such as blacksmiths, coppersmiths, horse traders, or entertainers. In the case of Romania, which has the largest population of

Gypsies in Europe—between 1.8 million to 2.5 million people (out of a total of 8 million)—there are over thirteen tribes organized in this manner, and only the cortorari tribe, is "still nomadic and basically survive by scavenging from garbage dumps and by petty thievery" (Strom, 1993: 19). It is in part their nomadic life-style that first set the Gypsies apart, and as Angus Fraser noted in reference to the arrival of the Gypsies in Europe around the fourteenth century:

> settled people on the whole do not trust nomads; in European society where the majority were pressed into a life of piety, serfdom, and drudgery, Gypsies represented a blatant negation of all the essential values and premises on which the dominant morality was based.
>
> (as cited in Lewy, 2000: 2)

The term *Gypsies*, then, came to have a pejorative meaning historically, which much later prompted the adoption of the term *Roma* which "represents the new emerging ethnic identity of this population," a movement that started in the 1930s and asserted itself more firmly in the 1990s (Achim, 2004: 1). In this text, both terms will be used in compliance with the historical context within which these people were viewed.

Their origin and their migration: For centuries it was believed that the Gypsies originated from Egypt, which accounts for the similarities in their associated given names in various countries throughout Europe such as Gitans in France, Gitanos in Spain, and Egiftos in Greece. This assumption held sway from their first appearance in Europe until the 1783 publication of the first modern scientific work on the Gypsies, entitled *Die Zigeuner*, by German scholar H.M.G. Grellmann. Based on earlier studies in linguistics by Hungarian theologian Istavan Wali, Grellmann was able to demonstrate unequivocally that the spoken language of the Gypsies, Romani, was in fact related to Sanskrit, and was then able to situate the origins of the enigmatic nomads in India (Stewart, 1997: 27). This claim has since been substantiated by more recent research in modern genetics which has provided "unambiguous proof that all Roma are descended from a single founding population, originating from the Indian subcontinent around 40 generations ago" (Kalaydjieva et al., 2005: 1084). With Romani clearly established as an Indo-European language, it has been possible through the use of linguistics to "reconstruct in broad lines the itineraries followed by the Gypsies" migrating Westward from India, with the understanding that the migration into Europe "took place between the ninth and fourteenth centuries in a number of waves" (Achim, 1998: 7–8).

The reasons for the Gypsies' migration out of India are speculative and largely unknown given the absence of written evidence in reference to these nomadic people prior to the fourteenth century. Some historians have suggested that they were taken as slaves by Mahmud of Ghazni around the tenth century during the expansion of the Ghaznavid Empire into India, and as a result, the Gypsies eventually found their way into Afghanistan, Persia, and Byzantium and finally in Europe (Shastri, 2007). As the Gypsies migrated Westward, it is believed that there were two broad strands of migration: one over land heading through Byzantium and eventually passing through Thrace, with another travelling along the shoreline of the Middle East and entering Egypt via the Sinai (Strom, 1993: 10). According to historian Nicolae Iorga, the Mongol invasions into Eastern and Central Europe led by Genghis Khan and later Tamerlane are responsible for the arrival of the Gypsies into this region, and as slaves of the Mongol military they were later abandoned once the defeated armies retreated (Crowe, 1994: 107). This theory has been contested by studies conducted by Franz Miklosich who underlined the differences between the Tartar (Mongol) slaves and those of Gypsy origin, arguing that because the former were kept in fixed dwellings and had Turkic names in comparison to the latter which had Romany names and lived in tents, their arrival into Europe necessarily occurred at different times (Achim, 1998: 16). What is clear, however, is that by the late fourteenth century ample references can be found regarding the Gypsies in Romania who lived as slaves and were considered the property of the church, the state, or wealthy landowners and businessmen.

In the principalities of Wollachia and Moldavia, which would later become part of modern day Romania, Gypsy slaves worked as craftsman, blacksmiths, or entertainers and became the Romanian working class alongside the peasant farmers and local artisans. It was first recorded in 1385 that forty Gypsy families were awarded to the Monastery of St. Anthony in Vodita by Prince Voivide. Later, in 1445, it was documented that Prince Vlad Dracul of Wollachia brought back from Bulgaria "11,000 to 12,000 persons without luggage and animal, who looked liked Egyptians"; while later yet, in 1471, Prince Stephen of Moldavia returned from Wollachia with 17,000 Gypsy slaves to be incorporated into the labor force (Crowe, 1994: 108). In Transylvania, which was under Hungarian rule, Gypsies were not kept as slaves, which over time led to a large number of them abandoning their nomadic traditions and leading more sedentary lives as a natural social course of evolution (Achim, 1998: 20). This is an important point to consider when examining the current living conditions of many of the modern-day Roma in Romania whose history draws upon over four centuries of slavery which contributed not only to a protraction of a nomadic way of life, but also helped maintain their status as deeply impoverished social outcasts living on the margins of society. The emancipation from slavery that occurred on 26 August 1864 triggered an unparalleled Roma exodus out of the new Romanian Kingdom largely out of fear of re-enslavement. However, with no money, land, or resources, in addition to a ban on nomadism that soon followed, "the plight of Romania's Gypsies improved little because of emancipation," and in time and out of desperation, many of the Roma "offered themselves for resale to their previous owners" (Crowe, 1994: 121). Though it is clear that freedom from slavery marked a vital step forward for the Roma, their continued low socioeconomic standings within Romanian society would persist throughout the twentieth century.

Following WWI, when Romania's national boundaries now included Transylvania and Bukovina, its population more than doubled to 16 million, and Romanians now represented only 70 percent of the population, as opposed to 92 percent prior to 1918. This major demographic change over a relatively short period of time helped foster a sense of growing unease with respect to ethnic minorities in Romania (Sanborne, 1996: 37). At the time, the Gypsy population accounted for approximately two percent of the total population, or about 350,000 people, and the majority had "abandoned their traditional way of life, living instead among the Romanian population," all the while maintaining their marginal social status and their specificity of trade (Achim, 1998: 148). The issue of nomadism resurfaced within this context of changing ethnic composition, and unsuccessful attempts were made to forcibly resettle the Gypsies and to transform them into wage laborers. In the rural and urban communities within which they lived, Gypsies remained excluded from the majority population and "due to their marginal social position, poverty, high level of criminality etc., the Gypsies were regarded as a 'plague' for Romanian society" (Achim, 1998: 164). By the 1940s, growing intolerance for the Gypsy people resulted in the deportation of 24,686 nomadic and seminomadic Gypsies to forced labor camps in 1942, over half of whom died of starvation and disease (Achim, 1998: 169,172).This event paralleled Nazi Germany's final extermination policy toward the Gypsies who were seen as an undesirable and inferior race whereby "more than half a million Rom had been systematically murdered," accounting for more than half of the entire Gypsy population living in Europe at the time (Strom, 1993: 12). Once WWII came to end, Romania would soon become a part of the Warsaw Pact, and it is within the Communist era that ensued that considerable resentment and animosity toward the Gypsies was further enflamed and became more entrenched by the late 1980s.

Early Communist leaders in Romania adopted a strategy of assimilation and sedentarization with respect to the Gypsies. Dictator Nicolae Ceauşescu, who came to power in March of 1965, pursued this policy with fervor and strove to absorb the Gypsy minority into the working class up until the fall of his regime in 1989. It was felt that "although the anarchic and unproductive Gypsy way of life might have been a rational response to extreme social marginalisation and poverty . . . communist society could provide a home for the Gypsies and so integrate them into 'normal life'" (Stewart, 1997: 6). The allocation of housing for the Gypsies in rural and urban settings was in keeping with the belief that "the very existence of the Gypsy minority could be 'solved' by dispersing them among reluctant white communities," when in fact, it helped contribute to the ethnic tension between Romanians and Gypsies which reached back for generations (Fonesca, 1995: 150). In the 1980s, Ceauşescu agreed to allow Romanians of German descent, who were living in Transylvania, to emigrate to Germany for the sum of 10,000DM per person, leaving entire villages of homes vacated which were subsequently assigned to Gypsy families (Rady, 1992: 147–148). Such acquisition of state housing further helped reinforce the perception within the majority population that the Gypsies were in essence "harvesting wealth without having sown its seeds" (Stewart, 1997: 19), a sentiment that also extended to the social benefits received by Gypsies, who in general "regarded employment in a regular job as an imposition and gave the authorities a great deal of trouble" in their attempts to tie them to jobs (Achim, 1998: 195). The end of the Ceauşescu's notorious regime in December 1989 brought with it economic upheaval and political instability and unleashed widespread public hostility toward the Gypsy people, bringing to light human rights violations that would eventually catch the attention of the international community.

The majority of the Romanian population felt strongly that the Gypsies had profited greatly under the much-despised repressive communist regime, and as a result, they felt justified in exacting indiscriminate violence upon them. Houses were burned, families were evicted, and "organized attacks on Gypsy communities throughout Romania prompted thousands to flee the country, mostly to Germany" (Sanborne, 1996: 104). Helsinki Human Rights Watch reported that the "Gypsy population was an increasingly frequent target of discrimination and violence" (Helsinki, 1990), and protested the "pogroms against Gypsies in Romania" in a report published on 31 May 1991 (Crowe, 1994: 146). Economically, the Gypsies suffered acutely from the collapse of the communist regime, in part because their livelihood depended largely on benefits and subsidies provided by the state. As the Romanian economy continued to falter, many Gypsy families did not have any land to reclaim under land reform initiated by the newly elected government and "they also had no legal grounds to retain their houses . . . leading to the expansion of ghettos with all their attendant social consequences" (UNDP, 2002: 15). It became abundantly clear that the Gypsies occupied the bottom rung of the social and economic ladder in Romania, and given their degree of marginalization, low level of education, and growing poverty, their plight would only get worse unless a concerted effort was made to seek out a solution that took into account the complexities of their plight. The possibility of accession to the European Union (EU) would provide the impetus needed to motivate government leaders and international bodies to develop a strategy of inclusion.

On October 1993, Romania was admitted to the Council of Europe, a first step to achieving entry into the EU, and criteria was put forward by the European parliament that needed to be met within a given time frame for full accession. It is worth noting that Romania was the last of the former East Bloc nations to join the council primarily due to its ill treatment of the Magyar minority of Hungarian descent, as well as the ongoing human rights violations against the Gypsies (Sanborne, 1996: 137). Recognizing that Romania's economic and social prosperity depended largely on inclusion into the EU, President Iliescu vowed to reject any manifestation of racism, anti-Semitism, or any form of intolerance based on ethnicity or religion, and to address the problem of exclusion with the Gypsies, now referred to as the Roma. A first step in addressing the problems within the Roma communities, as well as in the larger Romanian society, was to conduct a preliminary study to obtain quantitative information that would enable policy makers to distinguish between stereotypical and oftentimes racially biased notions of the Roma and the reality of their daily lives. The University of Bucharest and the Research Institute for the Quality of Life published in 1992 the results of their study, entitled "The Gypsies Between Ignorance and Concern," which looked at quantitative data about the Roma that would help define their social and economic standings, as well as outline their level of deprivation and marginalization. The study reported that there were between 819,446 and 1,000,000 Roma, or between

3.6 and 4.3 percent of the population, living in Romania, with the vast majority, 79.4 percent, having no profession, and over half the families not having a single member employed in the workforce (Achim, 1998: 203–204). With such pervasive unemployment, it is not surprising to learn that 62.9 percent were living below subsistence level, in comparison to the national average of 16 percent, and that the projected trend was one of "a worsening situation of the Roma population at a more rapid pace than that of the country's population as a whole" (Achim, 1998: 207). To better comprehend their current low socioeconomic standings within Romanian society, it is essential to gain an understanding of how these marginalized people arrived at such a place to begin with.

The traditional nomadic ways of the Roma, in addition to their cultural predisposition for living without any strong attachment to the land and lack of concern for the accumulation of material goods and wealth, have certainly played a significant role in shaping the current living conditions of the Roma community. As Michael Stewart points out, it is important to dispel "romantic notions of the careless freedoms of caravans and campfires," and to recognize that though the "Gypsy's fantasy was that they lived easily and luckily . . . the reality was they lived in grinding poverty and were subject to multiple disadvantages" (Stewart, 1997: xiv, 25). Being accustomed to living on the margins of society, it is possible to see how since their arrival in Europe in the fourteenth century, the Roma have stood on the fringes of mainstream societies with minimal integration in part by their own choice to remain distinct, and in part due to the misgivings and mistrust of the majority populations of their host countries that kept them on the periphery. In the case of Romania, it could be argued that their unique history of having been kept in slavery for over four centuries helped determine their fate as a socially marginalized and excluded people. Though it is difficult to overstate the tragedy of this period in their history, it doesn't explain the commonalities of social exclusion and economic deprivation that are found throughout Roma communities of Central and Eastern Europe which did not practice slavery, with the exception of Romania. As the UNDP report "Avoiding the Dependency Trap" noted, "the weak social role of asset ownership, the provisional lifestyle strategies, and poverty facilitate[d] the Roma's social exclusion" (2002: 14), and in the context of a progressively industrialized modern economy, the Roma lacked the skills, education, and willingness to adapt to the growing changes within Romanian society in the 1990s.

When taking a closer look at the discrimination and social intolerance of the Roma by the majority population in Romania, it is possible to see a relationship between the resentment the majority population felt during the Ceauşescu era and the nation-building processes that took place after the collapse of the Communist regime. As mentioned earlier, it was widely believed that the Roma had profited unjustly from the benefits of the socialist system, and by all accounts, they were certainly the most deeply affected by the economic upheaval of the early 1990s given their level of dependency on state support. Michael Stewart (1997) explains that for the Roma during the Communist era, the state's "first sector earnings were less desirable than the second, private sector earnings, with self-employment in the second economy being more lucrative," with the Roma all the while reaping the benefits of a state-led economy (109). According to the UNDP (2002) report, this issue "goes far beyond social welfare: it is a key cause of ethnic intolerance and Roma exclusion." There was a pervasive belief among officials and the general Romanian population that the Gypsies "persist in retrograde traditions and mentalities, tend to lead a parasitic way of life, refuse to go to work and live in precarious conditions," and this belief would help shape the events that followed the overturning of Ceauşescu's regime (Crowe, 1994: 140). As Romanians sought to redefine their national identity, it invariably led "to ethnic intolerance because rejection of otherness is a major element of the nation-building process" (UNDP, 2002: 13) and the strongly felt resentment of the Roma, along with the violent outbreaks that ensued, only helped strengthen a sense of distrust and animosity between the Roma and the majority population. A solution to the problem would necessarily involve not only addressing the economic disparities within the Roma communities, but also the social component that would lead to a greater integration of the Roma into mainstream society.

As a follow-up to a 2003 conference on the Roma held in Budapest, nine Central and Eastern European nations, with the support of international organizations, initiated the Decade of Roma Inclusion 2005–2015, with the intention of finding lasting solutions to the socioeconomic problems faced by the Roma. This greatly impacted each nation as a whole. Recent data indicated that in Romania, 88 percent of the Roma lived below the national poverty line, the infant mortality rate per 1000 births was 18.6, and the under age five mortality rate per 1000 births was 22, the highest of all the nine countries surveyed. Equally alarming was the fact that "more than 40 percent of the children in Roma Romanian households experience severe under nourishment, bordering on starvation," and only 19 percent of Roma children were attending school (UNDP, 2002: 19,47,107). The Decade initiative, signed by Bulgaria, Croatia, Hungary, Macedonia, Montenegro, Serbia, Slovakia, the Czech Republic, and Romania, represents "an unprecedented political commitment by governments in Central and South-eastern Europe to improve the socioeconomic status and social inclusion of Roma within a regional framework," by addressing four main areas of concern, namely: employment, housing, health, and education (Decade Watch, 2005). Each nation is to develop an action plan that focuses on the Roma issues prevalent in their respective societies, all the while aligning their objectives with the United Nations' Millennium Development Goals (MDG) associated with their country. Though it is still early to assess the impact of such initiatives in any conclusive manner, it is possible to get an overview of the progress that has been made to date based on the publication of Decade Watch by Roma NGOs and activists who are supported by the Open Society Institute and the World Bank.

This report brings together research gathered from all nine participatory countries and highlights the progress that has been made to date, and draws attention to key areas that have not been addressed and are in need of attention. The authors emphasize that to date the "biggest gap in the Decade implementation has been lack of data on the Roma" covering the four areas of concern cited earlier, which echoes a point that had been raised in previous UNDP reports, and in particular in reference to the need for disaggregated census data (Decade Watch, 2007: 19). In the case of Romania, the study indicates that in the areas of education and health, there has been substantial advance made by the government, though housing and employment show less visible progress. The authors recognize the current segregated education system to be an acute problem in Romania, though they highlight as one of the key achievements for the country, important steps taken in desegregation and affirmative action mechanisms that are helping the Roma gain access to primary and secondary education. The area of housing, however, remains a contentious issue. Local authorities have continued to evict the Roma from their homes and relocate them on the outskirts of rural and urban centers. Such action propagates a "pattern of housing rights violations that further deepen segregation and marginalization," and "central authorities have made no effort to stop, reverse, or correct the actions of local authorities." This point underlines a crucial element that is essential to the successful implementation of the Decade proposal, and that is one of mutual trust. In essence, it requires overcoming patterns of social interaction and exchange between the Roma, the government, and the larger Romanian population that has been marked by mistrust for generations, if not centuries.

As Viorel Achim states, "we are dealing with a life strategy specific to a community that suffers discrimination and marginalization, and that lives by the exploitation of marginal resources . . . making its social integration all the more problematic" (209, 214). The Roma representatives who participated in the declaration of the Decade of Roma Inclusion 2005–2015 have adopted a motto of "nothing about us without us" adding that "Roma participation will make or break the Decade." Certainly one of the more serious criticisms that appear in the Decade Watch report is that the draft version of the action plan put forward by the Romanian government involved no direct participation or input of the Roma community, nor the Roma NGOs representing them, which calls into question how Roma inclusion is to be achieved if they are not a part of the policy-making for this transformative social and economic process. The important issue of trust surfaced in the earlier UNDP (2002) report that stated how the majority of the Roma "have little trust of intermediaries such as informal leaders, NGOs, and political parties," adding that the local government has "a better chance for success at increasing confidence and trust" within the community. Given the abuses of power exercised by local authorities with respect to Roma housing, in addition to the lack of support from the national government on this issue, without forgetting the lack of inclusion of the Roma with respect to the agenda setting for the Decade project, it would appear that much work is yet to be done to build greater trust in order for the inclusion of the Roma initiative to succeed.

It is clear that addressing the problem of social exclusion, poverty, and marginalization of the Roma presents a formidable challenge for all parties involved. A long history of slavery, coupled by earlier nomadic ways of life, and decades of misguided attempts to assimilate the Roma into the majority population, in addition to choices made by the Roma to maintain a traditional lifestyle and to remain on the fringes of society, have all contributed to the present-day situation that sees the Roma as the poorest and most vulnerable in society. With Romania having recently been included in the European Union as of 1 January 2007, there is an opportunity for important social and economic changes to occur within the country that will help foster conditions favorable to greater inclusion and integration of the Roma into the larger society. Integration is in essence a two-way street in that "it requires changes both from majority populations as well as from minority groups, based on the understanding that integration (as opposed to exclusion or assimilation) is in the interest of both (UNDP, 2002: 4)." The persistence of patterns of exclusion with the Roma, in addition to the intolerance and violence that is directed to them from majority populations suggest "that some deep and fundamental issues so far have been neglected in approaching the Roma" (UNDP, 2002: 5,7). Therein lies the real challenge for those intent on reaching the objectives of Roma inclusion: addressing the deep, fundamental issues centered on trust and individual responsibility. The progress has been made in helping bring the Roma into the fold of modern society in Romania is worth noting, yet there is a need for more transparent, open, and inclusive dialogue if the Roma are to be fully integrated in society. As Romania continues to undergo its nation-building process, it can only be hoped that in time, the benefits of Roma inclusion will become more evident to the greater society. Until then, change is likely to come in incremental steps, but with the support of the international and European communities, this period in time holds great potential in seeing the Roma one day fully included in a stable and ethnically diverse Romanian society.

Notes

1. UN High Commissioner for Refugees (UNHCR), *UNHCR Eligibility Guidelines for Assessing the International Protection Needs of Asylum-Seekers from Eritrea*, 20 April 2011, HCR/EG/ERT/11/01, available online at: http://www.refworld.org/docid/4dafe0 ec2.html [Accessed on 7 October 2013].
2. Although Oceania comprises as many as 15 countries, such as Australia, Fiji, Kiribati, Marshall Islands, Micronesia, Nauru, New Zealand, Palau, Papua New Guinea, Samoa, Solomon Islands, Tonga, Tuvalu and Vanuatu, here only a selected countries are included.
3. Most Indigenous people live in New South Wales, followed by Queensland, Western Australia, and the Northern Territory. The NT has the highest percentage of Indigenous people among its population and Victoria the lowest. Most Torres Strait Islander people live in Queensland, with NSW the only other state with a large number of Torres Strait Islanders.

3 Globalization and Social Determinants of Health

The previous chapter has offered an analysis of the locations and sizes of Indigenous populations. This chapter analyzes social determinants of health (education, employment, poverty incidents, inequality, life expectancy and social status etc.) of Indigenous peoples and where they figure in terms of health in a global context. Globalization, a buzzword in the recent analyses of world affairs, refers to the process of increasing interconnectedness among societies such that events in one part of the world increasingly have effects on peoples and societies far away (Castles, 2002; Lawllen, 2004).[1]

Globalization has appeared in many different forms, affecting most of the people of the world. A lot of attention has been accorded to the extreme positive and negative impacts that globalization has generated. Similar results can be seen among the Indigenous peoples. Little is known about the influence of social determinants of health in the lives of Indigenous peoples. Yet, it is clear that the physical, emotional, mental and spiritual dimensions of health among Indigenous children, youth and adults are distinctly, as well as differentially, influenced by a broad range of social determinants. These include circumstances and environments, as well as structures, systems and institutions that influence the development and maintenance of health along a continuum from excellent to poor. The social determinants of health can be categorized as distal (e.g. historic, political, social and economic contexts), intermediate (e.g. community infrastructure, resources, systems and capacities), and proximal (e.g. health behaviors, physical and social environment).

This chapter grapples with the facts of health inequalities experienced by diverse Indigenous peoples in the world. The analysis includes the social determinants of health (SDH) across the life course and provides evidence that not only demonstrates important health disparities within Indigenous groups and compared to non-Indigenous people, but also links social determinants—at proximal, intermediate and distal levels—to health inequalities.

The Social Determinants of Health and Indigenous Peoples

The growing interconnectedness in a myriad of ways (trade, bilateralism, social and economic connections, geopolitics etc.) is often referred to as globalization.

This is, of course, a process that has brought the world's people closer to each other. Globalization processes, characterized by the increasing circulation of peoples, ideas and commodities, prompt the emergence of organizational forms that are intended to control, adapt and tap into those circulations. Thus, "many of the functions held by the nation-state are transferred upwards to supranational institutions and common markets through economic and political integration, downwards to regions and communities through political and administrative decentralization, and sideways to NGOs and the private sector through 'democratization' and privatization" (Blaser et al., 1997: 223–226).

Globalization might have profoundly deleterious effects on some states and may well increase inequality among them. As globalization has not impacted equally all the regions of the world and the Indigenous community has often been ignored, there is no doubt that globalization has not resulted in improved health in most cases of the Indigenous population (Kunitz, 2000: 1531). Arguments remain that globalization has positively affected the lives of Indigenous people. The question is how equitably globalization has impacted populations. For example, the Bangladeshi Indigenous population constitutes one percent of the total population in a major Hill Tract area. However, this area has been an isolated region for centuries. They have been kept aside from mainstreaming development, although some limited initiatives have been underway after a 1997 treaty between the government and the leaders of the local Indigenous population (Tebtebba, 2004). The major areas where the Indigenous live are highly militarized, which disrupts their lives.

In many independent countries, Indigenous and other tribal and semi-tribal populations are not yet integrated into the national community and their social, economic or cultural situations hinder them from benefiting fully from the rights and advantages enjoyed by other elements of the population (ILO, 1957). Thus, Indigenous peoples continually find themselves subordinated within the nation-state and international system (see Stavenhagen, 1996; Tully, 2000; Blaser et al., 2008). Therefore, in many cases, the status of the Indigenous people could be characterized as being marginalized and isolated from mainstream development when compared to other groups from whom they are distinct or when compared the nation-state as a whole, with limited participation and influence over external policies concerning their territorial, environmental and societal governance (Kearney, 1995).

During the twentieth century, Indigenous peoples were excluded from major decision-making processes and development plans. The Cold War also affected Indigenous people who were in the middle of ideological and armed conflicts in the region—Nicaragua and Guatemala, for instance (Lucero, 2001). Thus, in reaction to that history of abuses from the colonial empires, Indigenous peoples worldwide are struggling for political recognition. In this struggle Indigenous movements neither challenge the nation-state as a political community, nor democracy as a political regime. Rather, Indigenous demands challenge political institutions and their performance because those institutions have excluded them from decision-making processes (Warren, 1997).

Globalization has undoubtedly brought a lot of benefits for the Indigenous people who have been able to enter into new jobs and connect with outside world, however, for the very poor, the picture is not as promising. They are marginalized further by globalization while still being exploited by it. Globalization has accelerated the negative trends of economic and social development for the poor Indigenous people (Harcourt, 2001: 86) who have historically been the most vulnerable and most excluded ones in the world. They have faced serious discrimination in terms of their basic rights to their ancestral property, languages, cultures and forms of governance, but also in terms of access to basic social services such as education, health and nutrition, water and sanitation, and housing (AMAP, 1997).

However, the question arises: while globalists argue that the world is being benefited by globalization, how about the Indigenous populations? There are not many evidences that globalizations have not positively impacted on the life of Indigenous population. Some elements of economic globalization are still forms of exploitation, and they exclude certain groups of Indigenous people from the benefit packages of development initiatives (Osman, 2000). At the same time, there are evidences that globalization has had both negative and positive impact on the social determinants of health (SDH) of the Indigenous people. Theoretically, fundamental issue of inclusion and exclusion is differentiating between the human groups. In the new economic order, Indigenous families break down and are replaced by participation in national and international markets. Individuals who possess the characteristics necessary to "fit into global markets, whether for labor, capital or cultural goods, are included into the global order as citizens, with civil, political and social rights" (Castles, 1998: 179).

Therefore, evidence is not rare that Indigenous populations have also been excluded from the specific basket of basic services, especially health services. As a result, the health of Indigenous people worldwide is much worse than that of other communities—even the poorest communities in the countries where they live. The relatively poor health of Aboriginal people in the North America, Latin America, Oceania and Asia has been well documented. However, studies find that Indigenous communities are even worse off than other poor people in Asia, Latin America and Africa, as well. Looking at infant mortality among the Nanti tribe in Peru, the Xavante in Brazil, the Kuttiya Kandhs of India and the Pygmy peoples of Uganda, researchers found much worse figures than in the "host" communities (BBC, 2006). In Asia, especially in Bangladesh, they have only recently received the attention of development interventions. For example, the treaty between the government and the leaders of the Indigenous peoples in Chittagong Hill Tracts has brought them the possibility of development interventions and health services.

The major contributing factors to the poor health of the Indigenous population are: social factors such as dispossession, dislocation and discrimination; disadvantages in education, housing, income and employment; and physical environmental factors (Ullah and Routray, 2007). The social, economic and environmental disadvantages underlie specific health risk factors, and often contribute to lack of access to good quality health care (Australian Bureau of Statistics, 2004; Freitas et al., 2004). Industrialized societies have undergone various transition stages that involve a change from receding pandemics to lifestyle diseases. The pattern seems to be similar in Indigenous people in their traditional lands, such as the Pacific, and in newly adopted metropolitan centers, such as New Zealand. These are linked to socioeconomic transitions beyond their power and their borders (Fidler, 2001; Xanthaki, 2002; Carino, 2005).

Lucas (2005) argues that the free-market, neoliberal economic model and globalization are the cause of many health problems. These include the indiscriminate use of toxic products in agriculture, pollution caused by the oil industry, the consumption of transgenic crops, the destruction of the urban environment by pollution, and the commercialization of health services.

It is well known that Indigenous people are in an inferior economic and social position vis-à-vis the non-Indigenous, or "mainstream," population. Globalization is one of the key challenges facing health policy makers and public health practitioners (Dyck et al., 2002). Although there is a growing literature on the importance of globalization for health, there is no consensus either on the pathways and mechanisms through which globalization affects the health of Indigenous populations (Bird, 2002; Crowshoe, 2005). WHO identifies some of the most important social determinants of health (Wilkinson and Marmot, 2003).

> Social determinants of health (SDH) are the economic and social conditions that influence the health of individuals, communities and jurisdictions as a whole. Social determinants of health determine whether individuals stay healthy or become ill (a narrow definition of health). Social determinants of health also determine the extent to which a person possesses the physical, social and personal resources to identify and achieve personal aspirations, satisfy needs and cope with the environment (a broader definition of health). Social determinants of health are about the quantity and quality of a variety of resources that a society makes available to its members.
>
> (Raphael, 2004: 1)

Laura Alfaro (2004) argues that by generating increasing unemployment, poverty and rural migration, the "capitalist economic model" is the main cause of the return of illnesses that had been basically eradicated and of deaths from easily curable ailments. Rural and urban families are forced to live in overcrowded conditions without piped water or plumbing, to share collective bathrooms, and to live under roofs of corrugated iron or cardboard (Carino, 2005). Income levels among the Indigenous group, as well as human development indicators such as education and health conditions, have consistently lagged behind those of the rest of the population. According to Raphael (2004), education, employment, poverty, economic inequality and social status are the primary SDH. The following section sheds light on these variables.

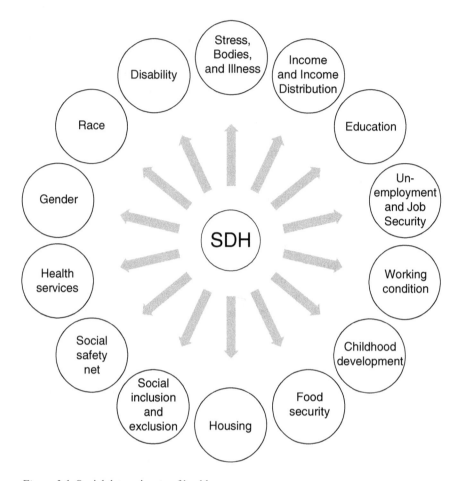

Figure 3.1 Social determinants of health

A Framework with SDH

SDH are the "fundamental structures of social hierarchy and the socially determined conditions in which people grow, live, work and age" (WHO cited in
KAHR, 2008: 1). However, social and economic circumstances determine the
health access, behaviors and health status of an individual. Under-allocation for
health care for Indigenous peoples is common (KAHR, 2008). About 80 percent
of the Indigenous populations in the Americas rely on traditional healers as their
primary health care provider (PAHO and WHO, 2006).

Education, one of the most significant social determinants of health, is associated
with economic growth, occupational specialization, and the emergence of services
that tend to be relatively egalitarian in organization (Ranger, 2003). Therefore, the
correlation between quality and levels of education of the Indigenous peoples and

their level of poverty is strong. Data show that participation rates for Indigenous secondary school students worldwide are significantly lower than non-Indigenous (Lehman, 2003). For example, in Australia, in 1996, nearly 11 percent of the Indigenous population held post-secondary qualifications, compared to 30 percent of the total population. In 1996, nearly half of Indigenous people of working age had no formal education in Australia. Although schooling in Australia is compulsory until the age of 15 years, participation rates by Indigenous primary students were lower (around 86 percent) than those for non-Indigenous students (about 93 percent). Indigenous people often have limited access to employment opportunities, which affects their motivation to remain in the education system beyond the compulsory years of schooling (Tse et al., 2005). The gap in the participation rates by Indigenous students in schools is even wider in developing nations. The public school system in Canada has been under stress in recent years due to budget cutbacks, labor conflicts and pressure to address increased needs, such as special education. If the universal system is not able to respond to such challenges successfully, an important pillar in the Canadian social structure will be threatened, which will have impact on the health of Canadian children (Ungerleider and Burns, 2004). In 2003, UNESCO convened a Ministerial Round Table meeting on Quality Education within the 32nd session of the General Conference to address one of the most elusive of the goals agreed upon at the World Education Forum at Dakar in 2000: quality education for all.[2]

Critics find both negative and positive effects of globalization on education of the Indigenous peoples. However, we argue that the impact on health of the poor is more severe, as globalization has led education to commercialization, which has limited the access poor Indigenous peoples have to education. Though the claim is that today education has become more efficient by the market force, it is moving away from the traditional concept of education as a publicly provided social good. Neoliberalism—that government regulation and the public sector should both be as minimal as possible—is not unique to debates over education. In the neoliberal model, making education commoditized has had more impact on the Indigenous population, as the poor have less access to education.[3] These contemporary world affairs have also contributed to education; however, a wide array of Indigenous populations have been left aside from the benefits of globalization. Available evidence of structural discrimination against Indigenous people takes the form of marginalization, exclusion and poverty and places Indigenous people systematically in the lowest income quintiles in many countries, mostly in Asia (WHO, 2006).

Despite the fact that there are benefits of globalization and freer trade, in terms of improved allocation of resources and consequent gains in productive efficiency and economic growth, it has been blamed for a host of ills, such as rising unemployment and wage inequality in the advanced countries, increased exploitation of workers in developing countries and the de-industrialization and marginalization of low-income countries. Free trade has made the countries without strong industries compete with industrialized countries. Thus, the employment market has become more competitive. Therefore, Indigenous peoples with low skill and education lag far behind in the competition. Consequences are evident that along with many poor non-Indigenous societies, a lot of Indigenous societies in many countries have failed to compete with the developed countries, resulting in widespread unemployment and frustration; thus, their livelihoods became uncertain (ILO, 2001). Access to job opportunities has been limited for some other reasons such as a skewed job structure in communities; low education levels; lack of information about jobs available; unsuitable training programs; problems with labor services; a shortage of child care services; and discriminatory behavior. Scarcity of jobs and the resulting high unemployment rate are the major obstacles to improved employability among Aboriginal people, especially the women.

In Canada, rapid growth of the Indigenous population and the predominance of young people (56 percent of the Aboriginal population is under the age of 24, compared with 35 percent of Canada's population) are placing considerable pressure on the job market. It is estimated, in fact, that some 80,000 jobs are now needed to meet current demand, and about 15,000 more jobs will be required every year to absorb young Aboriginal workers entering the labor market (ILO, 2008). By 2015, some 62 percent of the Aboriginal populations reached working age, which was barely 53 percent in 1996. Furthermore, since the mid-1990s, government's role has been changing, partly through budget constraints and public service job cuts. Several studies have revealed that these measures exacerbate the unstable working conditions of Indigenous women, directly contributing to greater poverty among them (Statistics Canada, 1993; MSRQ, 1995; RCAP, 1996). Aboriginal women living in cities are affected even more than the men by the scarcity of jobs due in part to the gradual disappearance of various occupations in the service sector (RCAP, 1996).

We can observe the disparity in labor force participation between Indigenous and non-Indigenous if we take one of Canada's provinces as an example. The labor force participation rate for Aboriginal people in Quebec is around 54 percent, while it exceeds 62 percent in the rest of the country (DIAND, 1996). Despite being generally more educated than men, fewer Aboriginal women hold a job (47.1 percent female and 57.1 percent male). This disparity (10 percent) between men and women is smaller, however, than that observed elsewhere in Canada among the non-Aboriginal population (15 percent) (DIAND, 1996). Aboriginal women also post a lower unemployment rate (17.7 percent) than their male counterparts (20.8 percent)—unlike in the rest of Canada. This is attributable to the fact that Aboriginal women enter the labor force less often than men, seek a job less often and are less available for a job than their male counterparts because of their role in the family. Their low unemployment rate suggests greater ease in finding a job when they return to the labor force and a tendency to keep their jobs longer (RCAP, 1996). However, evidence suggest that Indigenous peoples are subject to health hazards when they are employed—and unemployed, as well—although this picture might be different across countries. Although a job may offer access to health services, stress at work is often detrimental to health. Work is often associated with increased risk of low back pain, cardiovascular disease and depression (Wilkinson and Marmot, 2003). The argument is that Indigenous peoples have little control over their work, which further means that they are often offered jobs in the lower rung of the hierarchy. Statistics Canada (1999) found that twenty-six percent of married fathers, 38 percent of married mothers, and 38 percent of single mothers report severe time stress, with levels of severe stress rising by about 20 percent between 1992 and 1998 in Canada. At the same time, unemployed people and their families experience great psychological and financial problems and they are substantially at increased risk of premature death (Wilkinson and Marmot, 2003). Again, job insecurity has been shown to increase depression, anxiety and heart disease. Only one-half of all working Canadians have a single, full-time job that has lasted six months or more (Polanyi et al., 2004).

In Australia, labor market interventions such as government services and programs variously aimed at increasing the economic and social participation of Indigenous people include the Community Development Employment Projects (CDEP) and the Job Network. CDEP is central to the lives of many Indigenous people and is their main connection with employment of any kind. Throughout Australia, around 25 percent of all Indigenous employment is accounted for by the CDEP (Polanyi et al., 2004). The Job Network is the Commonwealth's employment and training provider organizations. The Network is made of independent organizations who are contracted by the Commonwealth to provide employment services to job seekers. CDEP provides employment for Indigenous people in a wide range of community projects and enterprises, and assists Aboriginal and Torres Strait Islander communities and organizations to take control of their own communities' economic and social development (Arbon et al., 2005: 68).

Poverty has profound effects on Indigenous health. Regardless of how to measure health outcomes, there is no doubt that poverty leads to ill health. Health outcome measures include: subjective self-reports, mortality, emotional stability, chronic conditions, general life satisfaction and physical functioning (CICH, 2004). In addition to the direct effects of being poor, Indigenous health can be compromised by living in neighborhoods with high concentrations of unemployment, poor housing, a poor environment and limited access to services (Wilkinson and Marmot, 2003).

In general, Indigenous Peoples often are more vulnerable to poverty than non-Indigenous peoples. The magnitude of poverty and degree of disparity are surprising. If measured in absolute terms, a person living in poverty lacks the means to buy goods and services designated as essential (Fellegi, 1997; HRDC, 1998). Research focusing on individuals has found a robust relationship between an individual's income and that individual's health, using a range of measures for both. Over the past 30 years, much research has contributed to understanding Indigenous peoples' culture and their health issues. Researchers such as Eastwell (1977), and Gracey (1983) have outlined both Indigenous and non- Indigenous people in understanding Aboriginal health (Shah et al., 2003).

An unfair ratio exists; for example, Indigenous populations constitute 5 percent of the world's population, yet they account for 15 percent of the world's poor and they account for approximately one-third of the world's extremely poor rural dwellers (UNPFII, 2014). The overall poverty rate among Indigenous families is almost three times higher than among non-Aboriginal families worldwide (Tse et al., 2005). Furthermore, during the mid-1908s, half of all Indigenous children were living in poverty, more than two-thirds were in near poverty (income below 120 percent of the poverty line) and one-fifth was in severe poverty (income below 80 percent of the poverty line) (Walker and McDonald, 1995). Income is a significant indicator of SDH and the resources on which living standards depend. Many of the disadvantages Indigenous people face are directly related to the low incomes.

Some have wondered if there is a way out to get rid of this poverty trap among Indigenous people (Freitas et al., 2004). Poverty reduction among Indigenous people is not simply a matter of service delivery; rather, it is about equipping them with the capabilities they need to lead the kind of life they value, to be free from fear and to enhance their role as agents in transforming their lives. However, living far from centers of power, it is difficult for them to influence the policies, laws and institutions that could improve their living conditions, including health (Freeman et al., 1992). This implies that their participation in the process is important.

The level of poverty of Indigenous people seems to be deeper as measured by the poverty gap—that is, the average incomes of the Indigenous poor are further below the poverty line (Kearney, 1995; Ullah and Routray, 2003, 2007). Plausibly, Indigenous poverty rates have declined more slowly than non-Indigenous because Indigenous people began at lower income levels. Where overall poverty rates were improving, income gains actually did not accrue equally for Indigenous people, as a result of low initial incomes, and fewer moved across the poverty line. The average amount by which a poor household's income falls short of the poverty line is also often reported. A number of researchers have argued that the intensity of poverty should be assessed by using a measure that pays attention to both incidence and depth of poverty as well as to inequality among the poor (Hye, 1996).

An example from the poverty situation of the Indigenous peoples in Australia is worth presenting. By all reckonings, Aboriginal and Torres Strait Islander peoples in Australia experience a disproportionate degree of poverty compared to non-Indigenous people. The indicators of Indigenous disadvantage are complex and interrelated. In the areas of health, education, housing and employment, Indigenous-specific programs exist; however, the funds are often insufficient to remedy the level of need or are inappropriately allocated (Xanthaki, 2002).

Evidence suggests that Indigenous people recover more slowly from an economic crisis. For instance, in Mexico, Guatemala and Bolivia, where national poverty rates have declined, the poverty gap,[4] as well as the poverty rate, shrank more slowly for Indigenous people relative to the non-Indigenous, and a similar situation prevails in Ecuador and Mexico (Xanthaki, 2002). In Mexico, in municipalities with a large Indigenous population, poverty is almost four times greater and extreme poverty is 20 times greater than in non-Indigenous municipalities. Although they enjoy a greater political presence today, a majority of the roughly 45 million Indigenous members of 400 ethnic groups found in the Americas, mainly in Bolivia, Ecuador, Peru, Guatemala and Mexico, remain firmly in the grip of poverty and marginalization (IPS, 1999; Crowshoe, 2005).

Moreover, gender issues further aggravate poverty among Indigenous peoples; for example, in Guatemala a non-Indigenous man can earn 14 times more than an Indigenous woman (IFAD, 2002b). There is no exception to this across the world. However, most countries have made little progress in addressing the issue of poverty among the Indigenous peoples. In 2000, 14.7 percent of Canadians were poor, which is a higher percentage than in pre-recession 1989 (around 14 percent). Seniors were the only group for which the poverty rate decreased during this period (moving from 22.5 percent to 16.4 percent) (Curry-Stevens, 2004). Child poverty in Canada increased during the 1990s, from 14.7 percent in 1989 to 15 percent in 2004, representing one in six children (Canadian Institute of Child Health, 2004; Curry-Stevens, 2004).

The impact of trade liberalization on the level of employment is an important determinant of its impact on poverty, wage and income distribution, and on the quality of employment (ILO, 2001). The increased trade between the advanced and developing countries has led to fears that increasing imports from low-wage economies, together with the relocation of labor-intensive industries there, were leading to serious job losses among low-skilled workers in the advanced countries in the early 1990s (ILO, 2001).

Economic Inequality

Economic inequality, referring to the gap between the richest and poorest in a society, may be a more significant social determinant of health (SDH) than absolute poverty. As mentioned already, there is a strong correlation between poverty and health, and as the gap between rich and poor widens, health condition worsens (Raphael, 2002; Auger et al., 2004). Income affects health in different ways; material deprivation—such as shelter and food—removes the prerequisites for healthy development. Participating in society while living on a low income causes psychosocial stress, which damages people's health, and low income limits people's choices and works against desirable changes in behavior (Curry-Stevens, 2004; Raphael, 2004).

With the lowest living standard in many countries in the world, especially in Bolivia, people have inadequate health, education, and social care. Half of the country's 9 million people survive on less than $2 a day; 30 percent on less than $1. Again, hardest hit are the nation's Indians, who comprise 60 percent of the population, giving Bolivia the continent's largest per capita Indigenous population (Curry-Stevens, 2004). This means that economic inequality between the Indigenous and non-Indigenous are even wider. Bolivia was dominated by the Inca Empire prior to the arrival of the Spaniards, who used the labor of the Indigenous population to search for mines. Pre-contact institutions were adapted by the Spaniards to benefit them in their efforts to use Indigenous labor. However, Bolivia's 1952 Revolution significantly changed the country's traditional order and the status of Indigenous inhabitants, and one of the most notable changes was the abolition of forced labor (Serafino, 1991).

Social and psychological circumstances can cause long-term stress to human health. Continual anxiety, insecurity, low self-esteem, social isolation, and lack of control over work and home life have powerful effects on health, especially on immune systems. People with less social standing usually run at least twice the risk of serious illness and premature death as those with more. This is an effect that is not limited to the poor, but extends across all strata of society, and Indigenous people are no exception (Wilkinson and Marmot, 2003). When measured by the other social determinants of health (SDH), such as poverty, unemployed Indigenous people were found to be far below the non-Indigenous (Wall, 1998). We generally tend to refer to socioeconomic status to explain health inequalities between Indigenous and non-Indigenous groups. Systematic evidence on health inequalities among the Indigenous still remains scant in most low income countries. The Indigenous have been, however, striving to develop a variety of ways to govern their own societies to keep their own traditional economic systems unharmed (Lasimbang, 2008).

Social exclusion denies individuals the opportunity to participate in the activities normally expected of members of their society. There is evidence of growing social exclusion in Canadian society, particularly for Indigenous people, non-European immigrants and people of color. Indigenous people are more than twice as likely to live in poverty and three times as likely as the average Canadian to be unemployed, despite their levels of qualifications (Galabuzi, 2004). Social isolation and exclusion are associated with increased rates of premature death, depression, higher levels of pregnancy complications and higher levels of disability from chronic illness (Wilkinson and Marmot, 2003; McIntyre, 2004).

Life expectancy, another significant social determinant of health status, has been reported dropping for the Indigenous, particularly for women, worldwide. Data show that in 1997–99, life expectancy dropped to 56 years for Indigenous men and 63 years for Indigenous women in Australia; during the period 1991–96, it was approximately 57 years for males and 66 years for females (Tse et al., 2005). Similar life expectancy rates have not been experienced in Australia by the total male population since 1901–10; by the total female population, since 1920–22. Life expectancy of Indigenous females at this time was comparable to that for women in countries of severe social crisis, such as Iraq, Western Sahara, and Pakistan, while Indigenous male life expectancy was comparable to that of men in Lesotho, Western Sahara and Bolivia (Australian Bureau of Statistics, 2002).[5] In Canada, research confirms that average life expectancy is five or more years less, and mortality rates are higher, for Indigenous people than non-Indigenous (Statistics Canada, 1998, 2000a; CIHI, 2000). Although the factors responsible for reduced life expectancy and higher mortality rates are diverse, one contributor is increased suicide rates; "Aboriginal status is associated with a 150 percent increase in risk of suicide" (CIHI, 1999: 304). Other reasons include higher incidences of disease. The prevalence of diabetes among Aboriginals is at least three times that of the general population (Health Canada, 1999). Data also show they are at particularly high risk of HIV/AIDS (Health Canada, 2000; Statistics Canada, 2000b).

Among Indigenous adults, the main causes of death in 1997–99 were heart disease and strokes, accidents, self-harm and assault, cancers, and diseases of the respiratory system (Australian Health Ministers' Advisory Council, 2011). For all causes of death, there were nearly three times as many deaths for Indigenous men and women as for non-Indigenous Australians. However, expenditure on health needs is much lower for Aboriginal and Torres Strait Islanders than for other Australians in the major federal government-funded health programs (Australian Bureau of Statistics, 2002). In Australia, among the Aboriginal population, infant mortality is also higher than the national average, although there is no up-to-date and consistent data on either Indigenous infant or maternal mortality. In the 1970s, the Indigenous infant mortality rate was over 80 deaths per 1,000 live births, and by 1981, it had fallen to around 26 deaths per 1,000 live births, a rate equivalent to that experienced by non-Indigenous Australians in the 1940s and 1950s (Walker and McDonald, 1995).

Again, the fertility rate for Aboriginal and Torres Strait Islander women is higher than the national average: 2.2 children compared to 1.8 for non-Indigenous women in 1996 (Alan et al., 2005). The maternal mortality rate for Indigenous women in 1994–1996 was 35 per 100,000 live births, more than three times higher than the rate of 10 per 100,000 for non-Indigenous women. In fact, according to the modeled estimates of the World Development Indicators, in 1995 the overall maternal mortality ratio in Australia rested at 6 per 100,000 live births (i.e. it is nearly six times lower than the Indigenous maternal mortality rate) (Mackay, 2002). In Bolivia, life expectancy is 61 years; child mortality is 67 per 1000 births, with 9 percent of children five years or younger malnourished; it is estimated that 85 percent of the population consume less than the 2200 calories recommended for daily intake (Gaviria and Raphael 2001). Since the colonial period, many Indigenous peoples in South East Asia, especially in Thailand and Central Africa, do not possess citizenship and national identity cards (Larsen, 2003; KAHR, 2008).

Indigenous People and the SDH

Health inequalities are experienced by diverse Indigenous peoples throughout the world. Health disparities within Indigenous groups are linked to several social determinants, such as education, income, employment, housing, racism, connection with land, colonialism, and access to services, at three different levels, which are: proximal, intermediate and distal.

Canada's original people consist of First Nations, Inuit and Métis people, with an overall estimated population of 1.17 million (Postl et al., 2010). The total fertility rate for the period 1996–2001 was 2.6 for Aboriginal women versus 1.5 for Canada. Thus, a high proportion of this rapidly growing segment of the population are children. As for death rates, Canadian data shows that for Inuit infants the neonatal is 5.8 versus a national rate of 2.8, post-neonatal mortality rate is 10.8 versus 1.7 and infant mortality rate is 16.5 versus 4.6 (Statistics Canada, 2010). Rates in First Nations communities are intermediate but still reflect a relative risk of two or more compared with the Canadian infant population as a whole. In the 1980s, Aboriginal children suffered from several diseases such as meningitis, respiratory syncytial viruses and smallpox. Other diseases like tuberculosis and hepatitis remain an issue till this day. Rheumatic fever has been more prevalent and more severe in Aboriginal children, and diabetes has increased significantly in Aboriginal populations. The rate of dialysis in the adult population increases annually; the relative risk of requiring dialysis is twice that in the Canadian adult population. In addition, obesity rates are also increasing. The health status of the community can be attributed to the effects of the social determinants of health on physical, emotional and spiritual wellbeing of individuals or communities (Postl et al., 2010).

According to the WHO (2011), the social determinants of health are identified as the following: social gradient, stress, social exclusion, work, unemployment, social support, and early life. Canadian determinants of health are: education, income and social status, social support networks, employment and working conditions, social and physical environments, personal health practices and coping skills, healthy child development, culture, gender, health services, biology and genetic endowment. While these determinants are relevant for Indigenous populations of the world, emerging literature indicates that there are some specific determinants of health that have particular relevance for the health and wellbeing of Indigenous peoples, and they are: cultural continuity, physical and social environments, self-determination, connectivity to land and reconciliation, history of health issues, and, finally, racism and marginalization. At the community level, health care providers have identified the key determinants of health as balance; life control; education; material resources; social resources and environmental / cultural connections; and inequitable access to health services, education, employment and social support networks. This last has a profound impact on the ability that Aboriginal people have, as individuals, to make decisions and control their lives.

Social determinants of health have been categorized as "distal" (historic, political, social and economic contexts), "intermediate" (community infrastructure, resources, systems and capacities) and "proximal" (health behaviors and physical and social environments), and research conducted by Reading and Wiens indicates that distal determinants have the most profound influence on the health of populations because they represent contexts that construct both intermediate and proximal determinants.

A collection of background articles prepared for the WHO Commission on the Social Determinants of Health provides insights into the impacts of distal determinants of health, such as colonialism, racism and social exclusion and self-determination. For Aboriginal people, colonization resulted in a loss of control over their destiny; inequitable access to educational models that promote confidence and self-esteem; and restricted access to opportunities for employment, economic development and self-determination. The proximal determinants of health reflect on the impacts of health behaviors that have the ability to negatively influence the lives of Aboriginal people. The physical environments of Aboriginal people are stressors from several perspectives: many First Nations, Métis and Inuit communities are geographically distant from urban or rural centers, with their desirable resources in education, training, employment and health services. Intermediate social determinants are the origin of proximal determinants and include health care and education systems, community infrastructure and cultural continuity. Social exclusion for Aboriginal people is a consequence of environments that allow racism through established systemic and indirect processes. As a result, access to culturally relevant and appropriate health services and education is challenging for Aboriginal people.

For many Indigenous populations, health is a communal concept, which has clear implications for understanding determinants of health. Spirituality, relation to the land, and identity are often connected within ideas of overall health, meaning all would have to be incorporated into a framework for determinants of health. Although differences exist between Aboriginal groups in Canada, there are also commonalities in recognized factors of health, including self-determinants, colonization and poverty (Dyck, 2008).

The literature scan revealed several key principles or beliefs to be embraced throughout the work of developing a framework of determinants. Those of particular relevance to Métis are as follows: holistic, intertwined and fluid determinants, wellbeing driven, and culturally/contextually relevant. In this context, intertwined refers to the interplay between all variables where none can stand alone. The central components found in the literature scan include: self-determination, colonization, spirituality, land, and culture and tradition. These themes or components are very meaningful to Métis and can be used to form the basis of a Métis health determinants framework. Self-determination is an ever-increasingly common health determinant for the world's Indigenous Peoples, as is the impact of colonization. Both have had, and continue to have, a tremendous potential in affecting the wellbeing and health of Métis in Canada. Spirituality, while a very difficult and heterogeneous matter for Métis, is still highly relevant to health and wellbeing. Spirituality is an important part of life for Métis, as it is with most Indigenous populations. As Métis are highly diverse, and since spirituality is highly personal, this may be a difficult determinant to adequately capture. It would be difficult to underestimate the importance of land to many Indigenous Peoples, with Métis as no exception. Even though many Métis live in urban centers, nearly all feel a deep connection to the land. Such importance to the population cannot be overlooked when examining wellbeing. Culture and tradition are similar to spirituality in that they are highly personal components with no uniform definition. It is not an easy theme to capture within health determinants; however, it is a necessary determinant for health (Dyck, 2008).

At the International Symposium on the Social Determinants of Indigenous Health (2007), it was demonstrated that the determinants of Indigenous health differ from those of the mainstream population. This is in part due to how health is conceptualized amongst Indigenous populations compared to Western definitions, but also that some of these previously cited mechanisms are actually identified as distal determinants. Since the social determinants of health themselves point to the very fact that the mechanisms that influence health are humanly factored, socially influenced and unequal, colonialism should really be allowed into the debate (Lang, 2001:162). This piece explores what it means to understand colonialism as a distal determinant of Indigenous health. There are and have been direct effects of colonialism or colonial policies on Indigenous health—for example, the introduction of contagious diseases like smallpox; the extinction of the Beothuk; or the gamut of negative experiences within the residential schooling system, to name a few. However, the above disparities also reflect the protracted effects of land dispossession and sedentarization on cultural continuity, access to traditional economies, as well as physical separation from mainstream monetary economies. In other words, these health gaps hint at the distal effects of colonial legislation. The WHO lists proximal determinants of health or what we see on the surface as follows: health behaviors, the physical and social environments; what diminishes capacity, limits control of material resources and exacerbates health problems. Intermediate or core determinants are what create these proximal ones. The former include such things as community infrastructure, resources, systems (labor and education) and capacities (Czyzewski, 2011).

The National Collaborating Centre for Aboriginal Health (NCCAH) defines distal determinants of health as "the political, economic, and social contexts within which all other determinants [proximal and intermediate] are constructed." Colonialism is the guiding force that manipulated the historic, political, social, and economic contexts shaping Indigenous/state/non-Indigenous relations and accounting for the public erasure of political and economic marginalization, and racism today. These combined components shape the health of Indigenous peoples. At the intermediate level, this occurs via the funding and organization of the health care, education and labor systems; as well as the extent to which Indigenous peoples can operate their environmental stewardship and maintain cultural continuity. Along with these intermediate determinants, proximal determinants are also subsumed under this larger structural reality: that at the root of these determinants is colonial relations—relations that have produced and reproduce unfavorable conditions and environments. These conditions and environments determine healthy behaviors, or lack thereof, physical environments, employment and income, education, and food security. These are not coincidentally some of the areas mentioned earlier where disparities can be seen between Indigenous and non-Indigenous populations. The structural and systemic contexts make for colonialism to be distal. Distal determinants are generally beyond the individual or community's control and are the causes of causes for unjust life situations for certain groups or people over others. Exploring colonialism as a distal determinant of health is linked to examining how current ideologies and historic events influence the health of contemporary Indigenous peoples (Czyzewski, 2011).

Although there is certainly a huge variance of mental health factors from one community to the next, overall, suicide rates are five to six times greater among First Nations on-reserve youth than the general Canadian population (Health Canada, 2013). And "the 1997 First Nations and Inuit Regional Health Surveys, conducted across Canada. Colonial policies have produced their own collective mental disease that affects Indigenous peoples today; however, the impacts of these policies are compounded by colonial mentalities that produce and reproduce detrimental discursive environments (Health Canada, 2013). Recognizing colonialism as a determinant of health involves questioning whether colonialism is a finished project, one of ongoing unequal relationships, but equally, whether these relationships have real negative effects on health. As a result, interpreting colonialism as a determinant of health is related to recognizing its influence on Indigenous lives as multifaceted. From a mental health perspective, colonialism can be produced and reinforced within Indigenous mental health discourses, but its effects can also be embodied as a reaction to contemporary political, social, economic situations and historically through trauma (Czyzewski, 2011:5). Addressing the ongoing effects of colonialism, decolonizing Indigenous mental health discourse and allowing for just and adequate control over key dimensions, such as health services, is inherently related to self-determination and thus improving health. Therefore, reducing and possibly eliminating health disparities would require policy that addresses the structural causes perpetuated by the general population and the government via transfers of power, and a sustained commitment to change from settlers, the various levels of government, and the Indigenous community (Czyzewski, 2011).

Media has been treating with high importance the recent news of the attempt at suicide of a number of Indigenous people in Canada. An Indigenous community in northern Canada has declared a state of emergency after 11 people attempted to take their own lives in one day. The Attawapiskat First Nation in Ontario saw 28 suicide attempts in March alone and more than 100 since last September, with one person reported to have died (BBC, 2016).

Canada's 1.4 million Indigenous people have high levels of poverty (Time, 2016). Their life expectancy is below the Canadian average. Attawapiskat First Nation has been isolated in Kenora District, northern Ontario, Canada. The former chief Theresa Spence had a hunger strike in 2013 to protest over the Canadian government not providing enough money, education and health care for the tribe. They had a state of emergency in 2011, the third in three years, due to low temperatures and insufficient housing, and in 2013 they accused Stephen Harper's Conservative government of being right-wing and racist (BBC, 2016; Time, 2016). Another Canadian Aboriginal community in the western province of Manitoba appealed for federal aid last month, citing six suicides in two months and 140 suicide attempts in two weeks. Suicide and self-inflicted injuries are among the top causes of death for First Nations, Métis and Inuit people (BBC, 2016).

The poor health status of the Aboriginal women due to inequities in the SDH in Canada is quite well documented. For example, in 2001 the Society of Obstetricians and Gynaecologists of Canada noted that lower quality housing, poorer physical environment, lower educational levels, lower socioeconomic status, fewer employment opportunities and weaker community infrastructure are primary reasons why they suffered from health problems. Aboriginal women are at higher risk for alcohol and substance abuse, mental illness, suicide, diabetes, cervical cancer, as well as more frequently experiencing deleterious circumstances such as poverty; alarmingly high rates of spousal, sexual and other violence; inability to access safe, secure, affordable, non-discriminatory housing for themselves and their families (on- and off-reserve, in rural, remote and urban settings); and barriers and lack of access to higher education, job training, employment, entrepreneurial loans and investments, and related socioeconomic opportunities.

For an Aboriginal woman, in particular, addressing her health status and rem-edying illness and disease means proceeding via a holistic approach: one which incorporates physical, mental, emotional and spiritual factors with her personal situation, nature and the environment, as well as her family, community and other relationships and societal settings and interactions. However, the lived experiences of Aboriginal women in the twenty-first century often impose disconnection, isola-tion and marginalization in and from their own communities, and in the broader micro- and macrocosms of Canadian communities and society (NWAC, 2007).

Indigenous Australians experience one of the highest levels of health inequality suffered by any group in a contemporary developed society. A significant body of research in Australia from the past two decades documents the relationship between socioeconomic inequality and poor health. In Australia, Indigenous pov-erty is widespread, deeply entrenched and probably underestimated. The relation-ship between Indigenous poverty and Indigenous poor health seems an obvious one. Both the poor socioeconomic position of Indigenous Australians and the deplorable state of Indigenous health are uncontested. However, the association between these two factors may not be so straightforward (Carson et al., 2007).

Assessing Indigenous poverty from a number of dimensions provides some idea of its broad and entrenched nature. First, from an income perspective, Indige-nous households are clearly disadvantaged. ABS (2005) data confirm that in 2002 the mean gross household income ($394 per week) was only 59 percent of that of non-Indigenous households. In addition, the income gap between Indigenous and non-Indigenous households is not decreasing. Second, while in developed nations such as Australia the relatively high standard of living means that poverty literature concentrates on relative rather than absolute measures of poverty, this concentration overlooks Indigenous poverty. In contrast to non-Indigenous Aus-tralia, a significant proportion of the Indigenous population lives in conditions that meet the United Nations' definition of absolute poverty: "severe deprivation of basic human needs, including food, safe drinking water, sanitation facilities, health, shelter, education and information." The prevalence of easily treatable dis-eases associated with inadequate basic sanitation and living conditions, as well as a lack of access to safe and reliable water supplies in many Indigenous com-munities, provides strong evidence for conditions of absolute poverty. Finally, the poor socioeconomic circumstances of Indigenous Australians do not appear to be improving. Key indicators of Indigenous disadvantage show that there was only a slight improvement across core socioeconomic indicators, such as unemployment rates, home ownership and rates of post-school qualification during the second half of the 1990s through 2002. An identifiable impact on poverty has yet to be seen (Carson et al., 2007).

There are considerable conceptual problems in applying standard measures of poverty to Indigenous peoples. The Indigenous population, for example, is much younger. Fifty-seven percent of Indigenous people are aged less than 25 years compared with 34 percent of the non-Indigenous population in this age group (HREOC, 2003). Indigenous household formation also tends to be different. Not only is the average household larger, with 3.5 people per household compared with 2.6 people in non-Indigenous households, but Indigenous households are more likely than non-Indigenous households to be multi-family households (ABS, 2003).

As well as being unequivocally poor by any measure, Indigenous poverty is different. For example, poverty in non-monetary spheres was endemic in Indigenous households, even among those who were relatively well off in terms of income and living standard. Household overcrowding was an issue for relatively advantaged Indigenous families, as well as those on lower incomes. Also, negative interactions between Indigenous people and the criminal justice system were a common feature of Indigenous life, regardless of household income. Members of high-income Indigenous households were nineteen times more likely to have been arrested than their non-Indigenous counterparts. Additionally, being dislocated from traditional lands was a common experience in Indigenous households, irrespective of income. While it makes theoretical sense for there to be a relationship between these two phenomena, as Morrissey (2002) notes, there is almost no evidence on whether the social gradient of health holds true within the Indigenous population. What little evidence is available indicates that any relationship between poverty and health for Indigenous Australians may differ from that for non-Indigenous Australians. Indigenous people had poor health across all income distributions, and high-income Indigenous families were nearly as likely to experience long-term health problems as low-income Indigenous families. For Indigenous people who live in regional and urban areas, the level of their personal income and self-assessed health status are positively associated. Though those who live in remote rural areas are quite different (Carson et al., 2007).

While there is good evidence that, by almost all indicators, Indigenous people are significantly poorer than non-Indigenous people, and this affects their health in a way similar to the non-Indigenous population, Indigenous poverty is also different from non-Indigenous poverty. The complex nature of Indigenous poverty means that, theoretically, existing non-Indigenous models of the social determinants of health can probably offer only a partial explanation of the interaction between Indigenous poverty and health (Walter, 2007; Reading, 2009). The social, political and economic consequences of being an Indigenous person in Australia add a dimension that cannot simply be plugged into existing mainstream models.

Aboriginal populations in Canada are defined constitutionally as First Nations, Métis and Inuit, and they are physically displaced people. The land is a fundamental component of Indigenous culture, and it is central to the health and wellness of Aboriginal societies. As a result, the physical displacement of Indigenous peoples from their traditional lands and territories, in Canada and around the world, has negatively affected the collective wellbeing of Indigenous populations. Loss of land is one of the most significant factors contributing to culture stress within Indigenous communities (Bartlett, 2003). The diet and daily nourishment of the Aboriginal groups prior to colonization was provided by the physical resources of their traditional territories (Richmond and Ross, 2009). Aboriginal communities are more likely to experience the adverse health effects of government decisions that can dispossess them of their environments than non-Aboriginal communities.

The direct link between the health of Aboriginal peoples in rural areas and their environment relates to traditional food consumption (Kuhnlein and Receveur, 1996). Given the relationships between Aboriginal peoples and their traditional lands and environments, the consequences of environmental dispossession have had disastrous implications for the health of First Nation and Inuit communities living in rural areas.

The determinants of health in rural and remote communities have been identified as balance, life control, education, material resources, social resources and environmental/cultural connections. The first five of these determinants map well onto those recognized by Canadian health policy (e.g. personal health practices and coping skills, education, income and social status, employment, social environments and social support networks).

The cost of rapid change in lifestyle has been very high. Many turned to alcohol, drugs and violence as a means of consolation. These behaviors have contributed to the declining quality of the social environment, which is being shaped increasingly by the despair of a lost way of life, widespread dependence on health and social services, and the negative health behaviors associated with living in poverty (Kaseje and Oindo, 2005). In the Aboriginal context, reducing health inequality in health policies, health programs and future health research on the SDH cannot advance without recognizing the complex historical, political and social context that has shaped current patterns of health and social inequality. The health of rural First Nations and Inuit communities are marked by significant upstream determinants. It is impossible to move forward without an appreciation of a determined effort to understand the mechanisms through which they operate to affect measures of population health (Richmond and Ross, 2009). Rather, reducing these inequalities requires an integrated approach that seeks understanding of various complex processes, including environmental dispossession, cultural identity, and the social determinants of health, and the ways these processes interact to shape health in local places (Ompad et al., 2007).

In addition, in Australia, land and access to the land is a key determinant of health and wellbeing for Aboriginal people. The systematic displacement of Aboriginal and Torres Strait Islander people from their land since colonization has engendered cultural disruption, social exclusion, increased feeling of stress, decreased sense of identity, political and social oppression and a loss of control over lives and livelihoods. In 1980s, in some countries in South Asia, such as Bangladesh, non-Indigenous people were encouraged to establish their habitats in 'reserve' areas for Indigenous population. This has as well disrupted the normal way of their life. Empirical evidences suggest that Aboriginal and Torres Strait Islander people live in overcrowded and unacceptable housing conditions, smoke tobacco, drink excessively, try illicit drugs and have poor nutrition. This means that these people live much of their lives in an environment affected and created by colonization (SACOSS, 2008). Many studies bear out that Aboriginal and Torres Strait Islander people in Australia have a greater likelihood of suffering from ill health than other Australians and as a result they die at a younger age, experience disability and a reduced quality of life at greater rates than non- Aboriginal and Torres Strait Islander people. The mean age for Aboriginal and Torres Strait Islander Australians was 21 years while 36 years for other Australians in 2001; the life expectancies of Aboriginal and Torres Strait Islander Australians demonstrate disparity: 59 years for males, 65 years for females, and the comparison to the average life expectancy rates for all Australians over the same period (77 years for males, 82 years for females) reveals an unacceptable disparity in health inequity in Australia (AHRC, 2008). The existing racism and discrimination that has accompanied colonization got to do with levels of stresses. There is no doubt that racism contributes to reduced or unequal access to employment, adequate housing, education, medical care, social support and social participation (Ullah and Huque, 2014). In addition, racism causes negative emotional reactions that contribute to stress and mental health. It is well researched that racism leads to the use of substances such as tobacco, alcohol and other drugs (Ullah and Huque, 2014; SACOSS, 2008).

There have been many useful experiential studies elucidating the link between the social contributors of health and negative health effects for the disadvantaged. Importantly, this disadvantage affects individuals not only from birth throughout adulthood, but it has also been linked to generational disadvantage. Recognition of the negative health effects of the social determinants of health is being embraced by government and is beginning to inform social and health related policy (Gore and Kothari, 2012).

Government got a role to play in ameliorating the social impediments of health and wellbeing. Holistic strategies need to be developed and implemented that seek to address the social inequity that contributes to both the social gradient and negative health effects. Through health promotion, a number of steps are being undertaken in South Australia to address structural inequality. However, as the experience of poverty is growing both nationally and in South Australia, this may result in further experiences of ill health amongst the most disadvantaged groups (SACOSS, 2008).

Little is known about the influence of social determinants of health in the lives of Aboriginal peoples. Yet, the physical, emotional, mental and spiritual dimensions of health among Aboriginal children, youth and adults are distinctly, as well as differentially, influenced by a broad range of social determinants.

Proximal determinants of health include conditions that have a direct impact on physical, emotional, mental or spiritual health (Krieger, 2008). For example, in conditions of overcrowding, which are most profoundly experienced among the Inuit people, children often have little room to study or play, while adults have no private space to relax (Reading and Wien, 2009). In many cases, these conditions act as a stressor, which increases the likelihood of behavioral and learning difficulties in children and adolescents as well as substance abuse and other social problems among adults (Ullah and Huque, 2014). Family violence experienced at one time or another by almost three-quarters of on-reserve First Nation women, has direct impacts on myriad of dimensions of health, especially women's health which results in negative impact on the physical and emotional health of children. Without doubt, health behaviors represent a well-recognized proximal determinant of health (Krieger, 2008). Among Aboriginal peoples, the most relevant health behaviors include the overuse or misuse of alcohol, which is related to increases in all-case mortalities, and excessive smoking, the health effects of which are clearly expressed in high rates of heart disease and increasing rates of lung cancer, and poor prenatal care as well as drinking and smoking during pregnancy are directly linked to poor physical, emotional, and intellectual development among Aboriginal children (Reading and Wien, 2009).

Physical environments play a primary role in determining the health of populations. Physical environments that are largely detrimental to health have been imposed through historic dispossession of traditional territories as well as current reserve or settlement structures (Porter, 1999). The most pervasive outcomes of these structures include substantial housing shortages and poor quality of existing homes. The Rural Aboriginal peoples face considerable food insecurity related to challenges acquiring both market and traditional foods. Poor sanitation and waste management, unsafe water supplies, and lack of community resources are evidently jeopardizing the health of Aboriginal peoples (Reading and Wien, 2009).

"Through colonization, colonialism, systemic racism and discrimination, Aboriginal peoples have been denied access to the resources and conditions necessary to maximize SES (Socioeconomic status) (Reading and Wien, 2009: 13)". Around the world, the high rates of unemployment, scarcity of economic opportunities, poor housing, low literacy rate as well as meager community resources are the obvious results of their limited access to resources. In Canada, Aboriginal people are less likely than other Canadians to participate in the labor force and are even less likely to be employed. For those who are in the labor force, the level of unemployment is between two and three times higher than it is for other Canadians (Ullah and Labonte, 2007).

There is evidence of inequities in the distribution of resources and opportunities to Aboriginal peoples in Canada. For instance, despite the growing number of Aboriginal peoples—particularly women—attaining post-secondary degrees, inadequate educational opportunities for most adults manifest as a lack of capacity to promote education among their children (Shanker, et al., 2013). An estimated 50 percent of Aboriginal youth is expected to drop out, or be pushed out, of high schools, resulting in diminished literacy and employment, as well as increased poverty in future generations (NCCAH, 2007). Poverty has outcomes on health because, in part, it determines what kinds of diet people consume and what they can afford to purchase (UN, 2009). Thus, persons at lower incomes are subject to the stress of food insecurity from a compromised diet that results when food is no longer available.

While proximal determinants represent the root of much ill health among Aboriginal peoples, intermediate determinants can be thought of as the origin of those proximal determinants (Krieger, 2008). For instance, poverty and deleterious physical environments are rooted in a lack of community infrastructure, resources and capacities, as well as restricted environmental stewardship (NCCAH, 2007). Likewise, inequitable health care and educational systems often act as barriers to accessing or developing health promoting behaviors, resources and opportunities.

The interaction of intermediate determinants is especially evident in the connection between cultural continuity and other intermediate determinants, all of which have a direct influence on proximal determinants (Greenwood and Naomi, 2012).

Current health care services focuses mainly on communicable disease, while mortality and morbidity among Aboriginal peoples are increasingly resulting from chronic illness. Reading and Wien (2009) go on to say that social access to health care is similarly limited or denied to Aboriginal peoples through health systems that account for neither culture nor language, nor the social and economic determinants of Aboriginal peoples' health. As with other Canadians, First Nation adults living on reserve have difficulty accessing health care services because of long wait lists and the fact that many First Nation adults live in rural and isolated communities got a number of economic barriers to accessing health care.

Adequate education has a profound impact on income, employment and living conditions. Well-educated parents not only earn higher incomes, thereby improving proximal determinants of health (Hye, 1996; Ullah and Routray, 2007), but they also pass the value of education and life-long learning to the next generation (Greenwood and Naomi, 2012).

The health of an individual and their family is substantially influenced by the community in which they live. However, economic development is a key determinant of health for Aboriginal peoples. Hence access to economic activities i.e. access to education and employment opportunities is important for them. Limited infrastructure and resource development opportunities have been important contributors to economic insecurity and marginalization, with subsequent deprivation among community members. In addition, inadequate social resources, in the form of qualified individuals who can develop and/or implement programs, restrict Aboriginal communities' access to funding (NCCAH, 2007). When communities experience fragmented, under-funded programs in which the bureaucracy increases community responsibility without a concomitant increase in power, community-level stress and paralysis can happen as a result.

Another key intermediate determinant of health that has been widely recognized is environmental stewardship. In fact, traditional ties to the natural environment are generally acknowledged as a major resource for the superior health enjoyed by Indigenous peoples prior to European colonization of the Americas. Unfortunately, the past 500 years have witnessed a rapid transition from a healthy relationship with the natural world to one of dispossession and disempowerment (Reading and Wien, 2009). Aboriginal peoples are no longer stewards of their traditional territories, nor are they permitted to share in the profits from the extraction and manipulation of natural resources. Finally, contamination of wildlife, fish, vegetation and water have forced Aboriginal peoples further from the natural environments that once sustained community health.

A landmark study of Chandler and Lalonde (1998) revealed that among First Nations people in British Columbia, rates of suicide (which are strongly linked to proximal determinants) varied dramatically and were associated with a constellation of characteristics referred to as "cultural continuity" (Reading and Wien, 2009). Cultural continuity might best be described as the degree of social and cultural cohesion within a community. Cultural continuity also involves traditional intergenerational connectedness, which is maintained through intact families and the engagement of elders, who pass traditions to subsequent generations.

Distal determinants have the most profound influence on the health of populations because they represent political, economic, and social contexts that construct both intermediate and proximal determinants (Krieger, 2008). In the case of Aboriginal peoples, although intra and inter-group differences exist, to a large extent, colonialism, racism and social exclusion, as well as repression of self-determination, act as the distal determinants within which all other determinants are constructed (Reading and Wien, 2009). Historical research clearly indicates a link between the social inequalities created by colonialism and the disease, disability, violence and early death experienced by Aboriginal peoples in Canada.

The impact of colonialism on Aboriginal peoples' relationship with the environment began with their dispossession of and displacement from traditional lands in the twentieth century (Oviawe, 2013). The political agenda of the twentieth-century colonial system was to assimilate and acculturate (see Castles, 1998) Indigenous peoples into the dominant culture. I think the most powerful way of assimilation was to send aboriginal children to the residential schools. These school system later was considered the vanguard of genocide and re-socialization of Aboriginal peoples and through these schools, culture, language, family ties and community networks were destroyed for generations of First Nations, Métis and Inuit children (Reading and Wien, 2009). The results have been devastating socio-cultural change among all Aboriginal peoples, including disengagement by many from their ancestry and culture

Racism and its subsequent social exclusion creates barriers to Aboriginal participation in the national economy. Without equitable distribution of the determinants of health, Aboriginal peoples cannot realize the same possibilities for health. Relegated to the bottom of the social hierarchy, Aboriginal peoples are exposed to health damaging intermediate and proximal determinants, which increase their vulnerability to illness (Reading and Wien, 2009).

Self-determination has been cited as the most important determinant of health among Aboriginal peoples (Greenwood, 2012; Reading and Wien, 2009; Shepherd et al., 2012). Self-determination influences all other determinants, including education, housing, safety, and health opportunities. In order to ensure the most favorable intermediate determinants of health, Aboriginal peoples have to be given equal access to political decision-making, as well as their lands, economies, education systems, and social and health services. Of course, unfortunately, this remains as a rhetoric. The colonial agenda rather has enforced unequal access to and control over property, economic assets and health services. In many ways, this restrictive structure has actually encouraged Aboriginal social, political and economic development that is not self-determined.

The evidence indicates that social determinants at proximal, intermediate and distal levels influence health in complex and dynamic ways. The individual and cumulative effects of inequitable social determinants of health are evident in diminished physical, mental, and emotional health experienced by many

Aboriginal peoples (Zubrick et al., 2004). Unfavorable distal, intermediate and proximal determinants of health are associated with increased stress though lack of control, diminished immunity and resiliency to disease and social problems, as well as decreased capacity to address ill health. The complex interaction between various determinants appears to create a trajectory of health for individuals that must be addressed through a social determinants approach.

The experience of Australian and New Zealand Indigenous peoples has been different in some fundamental ways. Despite these differences, Indigenous peoples in both countries systematically experience poorer health. Like I mentioned before, Aboriginal people have significantly shorter average life expectancies than many people in the developing world and of those Indigenous peoples of Canada, and the United States of America, and of the Maori of New Zealand. As for morbidity, Aboriginal people are about three times more likely to be admitted to hospital than other Australians. Non-communicable, chronic and notifiable disease all contribute to the greater burden of ill health experienced by Aboriginal Australians. Mental health, social and emotional wellbeing in Aboriginal populations are still poor compared to other Australians, the impact of trauma, grief, racism and violations of human rights issues largely unrecognized.

High rates of established behavioral health risk factors, such as smoking, substance [mis]use, exposure to violence in the home and in the community, lack of exercise and having body mass indices of greater than 30 (technically obese), are well documented in Indigenous populations. The loss of land and marginalization of Aboriginal people accompanied by individual and institutional experiences of discrimination and racism have placed heavy burdens of stress, alienation and loss of sense of control on many individuals, families and communities (Westerndesert, 2007).

A review of changes in socioeconomic status of Aboriginal Australians between 1971–2001 by the Centre for Aboriginal Economic Policy Research (CAEPR) found that there have been slow improvements since 1971 but that Aboriginal Australians are still disadvantaged in comparison to other Australians (Altman et al., 2008). Slow improvement in disadvantage indicates that broad policy setting may be suiting most of Australia, but when the differentials close at a much slower rate, we cannot afford to be complacent while systematic differentials remain. Aboriginal Australians are less likely to have equivalent levels of income, employment, education, or level of home ownership. Furthermore, intermediate social determinants like child abuse and neglect, domestic violence and high levels of inter-personal violence have been reported in many Indigenous communities and are often accompanied by alcohol and drug abuse. Aboriginal people are more likely to have contact with the justice system irrespective of income.

The living conditions for Aboriginal Australians in rural and remote areas remain a source of national shame with many communities living in extremely poor quality housing without access to basic infrastructure such as safe, running water, drainage, all weather roads and access to affordable, high quality food, particularly fruit and vegetables. There is a difference in life style between the rural and urban Indigenous people. As noted earlier, most Aboriginal Australians live in urban areas, but even in this setting their housing is more likely to be over-crowded and poorly maintained. There has been some recognition that housing for Aboriginal Australians needs to be differently designed to be compatible with family structures and lifestyle, but progress in changing housing design has been slow (Hunter and Schwab, 2003).

Health for Maori, the Indigenous peoples of New Zealand, is an important feature of the culture. There is no doubt that by most measures of inequality, Maori experience an unfair burden that stems from social, cultural and economic deprivation. While the Maori population has grown alongside that of the Asian and Pacific populations relative to the 'European only' population, they have fallen as a proportion of the overall population by 0.5 percent in ten years. As for the epidemiology of the Maori people, Maori can expect shorter life expectancy (even when adjusted for low income), fewer disability-free years, more preventable illness, a poorer prognosis for cancer when it is diagnosed and poorer access to health services (Pulver, Elizabeth and Waldon, 2015). This situation has existed for some considerable time. As for mortality, life expectancy for non-Maori, Maori and Pacific men in 2000/02 was 77.2, 69.0 and 71.5 years respectively (Westerndesert, 2007). Life expectancy for women was 81.9, 73.2, and 76.7 years respectively and as we consider how long a person could expect to live a healthy life, non-Maori and Maori women were 68.2 and 59 years respectively, and men were 65.2 and 58 years (Waldon, 2010). Access to culture, land and economic resources are priority determinants for Maori as they continue to negotiate to improve the provision of a wide range of services critical to health and economic investment. The government has been unable to address inequalities characterized by the limited quality and range of socioeconomic indicators available. When economic conditions led to higher unemployment in the 1990s, Maori carried the excess burden of morbidity. Intermediate social determinants for Maori are characterized by inequalities that have a negative health dividend—poor housing and overcrowding with disease (Pulver, Elizabeth and Waldon, 2015).

In conclusion, persistent differentials in health and socioeconomic status for the Indigenous peoples of Australia and New Zealand have their antecedents in the social and political context that characterized early stages of colonization when structural determinants of health and wellbeing were changed. There is evidence that over the past thirty years progress has been made to improve the social determinants of health of Australia's and New Zealand's Indigenous peoples. However, by many indicators, Indigenous health remains unacceptably lower and at levels experienced nearly a century ago by non-Indigenous peers.

Many of the factors that Aboriginal and Torres Strait Islander people identify as impacting on their wellbeing are examples of systemic or institutional discrimination, which occurs when policies and procedures, or laws, serve to disadvantage specific groups or limit their rights. While often viewed as neutral and sometimes acceptable, the application of beliefs, values, structures and processes by the institutions of society (economic, political, social) result in differential and unfair outcomes for particular groups. Policy and practices that discriminate unfairly in their effect, impact or outcome, irrespective of the motive or intention, amount to unfair discrimination. The National Aboriginal and Torres Strait Islander Health Survey (NATSIHS) 2004–05 reported that 11.6 percent of Aboriginal Australian respondents in urban areas and 13 percent in remote and very remote areas experienced discrimination (Zubrick et al., 2011). Systemic discrimination is thus measured by outcomes and results rather than intentions— it is not necessary to examine the motives of the individuals involved but rather the results of their actions. In addition, Aboriginal and Torres Strait Islander-identified risk factors include widespread grief and loss, child removals, unresolved trauma and cultural dislocation and identity issues. These determinants of wellbeing highlight how the cumulative and interrelated effects of determinants such as family violence, substance use/abuse and mental health disorders impact negatively on other aspects of life. Together these various findings create a composite picture of the risk factors influencing poor wellbeing. These are manifested in a range of conditions from anxiety and depression, through to serious psychological distress, depending on the frequency and intensity and range of stressors experienced by an individual or family or community as well as the existence of protective factors. Little work has been done to identify the factors that have helped Aboriginal and Torres Strait Islander people to survive several generations of trauma and extreme disadvantage. Aboriginal and Torres Strait Islander people have been forced to rely on each other, and the cultural, spiritual and other forms of support that are an integral part of the oldest continuous cultures on earth, to manage wellbeing in individuals, families and communities. Certainly, the interdependent nature of family, kinship and community connectedness found in many Indigenous communities appears to offer some protection and warrants further examination (Zubrick et al., 2011).

Notes

1. This view was firmly embraced by the world's leaders who gathered in the waning days of the Second World War to rebuild a viable international order. They knew how an earlier era of economic globalization, in some respects as economically interdependent as ours, eroded steadily before collapsing completely under the shocks of 1914. That global era rested on a political structure of imperialism, denying subject peoples and territories the right of self-rule.
2. The meeting concluded that education needed to develop responses to the diversity of needs. Special provisions, from language training to access to higher education, should be made for the marginalized: Indigenous, special needs rural, immigrant and refugee populations. Inclusiveness in providing access to languages was underlined with special attention to Indigenous students. A strategy of literacy in local languages was considered essential to ensure quality.
3. Water is becoming a marketable commodity or merchandise to which only those who can afford it have access, which will have a negative impact on the public health of a large part of the global population (Lucas, 2005:1). The effects of transgenic food crops and the introduction of genetically modified seeds are giving certain transnational corporations control over food production worldwide, as is already occurring in the case of soy beans. The global market for transgenic soy is the monopoly of a single company, the US-based Monsanto, which sells seeds that are resistant to its Roundup herbicide (Lucas, 2005).
4. The position of poor people from the poverty line.

5. According to the 2001 Australian census, about 40 percent of Indigenous people were aged less than 15 years, compared with 20 percent of non-Indigenous people. About 3 percent of Indigenous people were aged 65 years or over, compared with 10 percent of non-Indigenous people (Australian Bureau of Statistics, 2003 and 2004). In Canada, the percentage of the adult Aboriginal population with less than grade 12 education is consistently higher than that for the non-Aboriginal population, with the most noticeable gap being in Winnipeg, where over one-half of adult Aboriginal people do not have the minimum education for employability. In terms of higher education, urban Aboriginal people are not as well off as non-Aboriginals (Young, 2003).

4 Globalization and Self-Governance

The previous chapter analyzed the social determinants of health (SDH) of the Indigenous population. This chapter demonstrates the interplay of SDH and self-determination. While there is extensive diversity in Indigenous peoples throughout the world, all Indigenous peoples have one thing in common—they all share a history of injustice and deprivation: they have been denied rights, killed, tortured and enslaved. Throughout the world (most of North and South America and through much of the Third World) an overwhelming aggression—legal, physical and psychological—against the Rights of Indigenous Peoples by colonial powers and by other nations has taken place. They have been denied the right to participate in political system and governing processes of the current state systems. In many cases, they continue to face threats to their very existence due to systematic exclusionary policies of respective governments.

Indigenous self-governance has become a prominent issue worldwide over the past several decades. The emergence of self-determination of Indigenous peoples has sparked a great deal of debate within legal circles. The conventional sentiment is that colonial controls and the resulting abuse governments have heaped on Indigenous people for more than a century must be revisited. The movement toward Indigenous self-governance is intended to provide greater autonomy in relation to financial and legislative authority. Many have described the contemporary ideal of Indigenous self-government as parity among Indigenous, provincial and federal powers in Canadian context.

Indigenous peoples often are not able to participate equally in development processes and share in the benefits of development, and often are not adequately represented in national, social, economic, and political processes that direct development. It is neither desirable nor possible to exclude Indigenous peoples from development. Like mainstream populations—the group or groups in a country that are politically, economically, and culturally most powerful—Indigenous peoples have developmental aspirations. However, Indigenous peoples may not benefit from development programs designed to meet the needs and aspirations of mainstream populations, and may not be given the opportunity to participate in the planning of such development. There is increasing concern in the international development community that Indigenous peoples be afforded opportunities to participate in and benefit from development equally with other segments of society, and have a role and be able to participate in the design of development interventions that affect them.

The eight goals known as the Millennium Development Goals (MDGs) were set by the global United Nations conferences in the nineties. One may easily notice that in the MDGs, Indigenous peoples are invisible. It is surprising how this historically distinct section of the population has been overlooked. Since the 1990s, Indigenous activists, scholars and people at large have analyzed the shortcomings of the MDGs. They have come to the conclusion that the MDGs are not shaped within a rights-based framework, and they argue that development has occurred without recognizing them and without according due respect to their individual human rights (Cariño, 2005; Tauli-Corpuz, 2005). There is a basis to fear that this sort of negligence, whether deliberate or not, leads to further discrimination, impoverishment and marginalization. Poverty and rights are inextricably linked. One is lame without the other. Cariño (2005) goes on to say that governments speak of "poverty" while Indigenous peoples speak of "rights." Therefore, the MDGs must be grounded in an approach that is inclusive.

Globalization and Self-Governance

The conventional sentiment is that colonial controls and the resulting abuse governments have heaped on Indigenous people for more than a century must be rejected. The movement toward Indigenous self-government is intended to provide greater autonomy in relation to financial and legislative authority. According to Wall (1998), hope of a renewed relationship between Indigenous and non-Indigenous peoples lies in Indigenous self-government (RCAP, 1993).

Indigenous movements worldwide are shaping the public policies of many governments. Currently, the Indigenous movements are pushing for the respect of the principle of self-determination of the peoples, which implies the recognition of the Indigenous peoples as nations. Many challenges that Indigenous movements have been posed such as: the Indigenous proposals for public policy (Warren, 1997), the strategies for Indigenous mobilization (Lucero, 2001), the quest for self-determination and autonomy (Díaz, 1997), and the building process of new types of citizenship in the multicultural Latin American societies (Mattiace, 2000; Peeler, 2000; Postero, 2000). Indigenous peoples' struggles are now carried on within complex transnational networks and alliances that traverse the boundaries between the state, markets and civil society, including the environmentalist and human rights movements (Blaser et al., 2008).

For many people, globalization has often come to mean greater vulnerability to unfamiliar and unpredictable forces that can bring on economic instability and social dislocation. The Asian financial crisis of 1997–1998 was such a force—the fifth serious international monetary and financial crisis in just two decades (BBC, 2006). The principle of the right of peoples to self-determination has been present in international debates for almost a century, and the current claims to this right by Indigenous organizations are only the latest instance of its use in the expanding debate about human rights (WHO, 2006). The concept of self-governance has different implications in different contexts. For example, in Canadian contexts, self-governance refers to the power, granted to Indigenous people within boundaries of Canada, to govern certain activities concerning themselves, within the existing structures of Canadian government, and with accordance to the Canadian Charter of Rights and Freedoms. Indigenous self-government is the power of Indigenous peoples to govern themselves as nations. Much as the Italians or Israelis or Swedes govern themselves, First Nations People want the same recognition to govern themselves as members in the global community (Chapleaucree, 1996). In the last three decades, Indigenous peoples' struggles to keep control of their lives and lands have moved from being of concern only to themselves, and some specialists and specialized bureaucracies, to being issues of wide public awareness and debate in many sectors of society (Blaser et al., 2008).

The UN Permanent Forum on Indigenous Issues was established on 28 July 2000 by the Economic and Social Council (ESC) on the recommendation of the Commission on Human Rights with the aim to serve as an advisory body to the ESC, with a mandate to discuss economic and social development, culture, the environment, education, health and human rights. It represents an historic advance in Indigenous peoples' efforts to reach the ear of the international community and make their needs and concerns known (UN, 2005). The second session of the Forum, held in 2000 at the UN Headquarters, drew up concrete recommendations for the UN system for improving the quality of life of the world's Indigenous peoples. The recommendations emphasized children's education and that Indigenous languages, cultures and values would be at stake (UN, 2005).

The Forum has further stressed the importance of quality education in pulling Indigenous people out of poverty and preserving their cultures and knowledge systems. It was argued that educational level alone couldn't result in higher incomes; it should be accompanied by a higher quality of schooling in many Indigenous communities. The forum gathered some 1,500 Indigenous leaders, activists and representatives in the year's Forum to press on Indigenous people and the Millennium Development Goals of eradicating extreme poverty and hunger and achieving universal primary education (UN, 2005). Critics of current forms of Indigenous self-government view them as little more than convenient arrangements that allow them administrative responsibility for services that are ultimately controlled by the federal or provincial government. They argue that self-government is essentially glorified municipal government; arrangements are not equal in legislative and financial authority to the federal and provincial governments (Wall, 1998).

Indigenous Peoples and Self-Governance

While many scholars, academics and politicians have created definitions for the word *globalization*, most of them agree that it has both positive and negative outcomes, particularly concerning the issue of the Indigenous peoples and their long fight to earn their rights in the time of globalization.

Tavanti (2003) views globalization as a double-edged weapon, one side made up of the "declining capacity for collective action on the part of marginalized racial groups and classes in society," while the other "produces a process of social re-articulation in the creation of new strategies of resistance" (Tavanti, 2003: 2). While Cesarotti (2000) defines globalization in its simplest form as the "integration" of the nations of the world; this assimilation has come about through international agreements of trade, international and transnational organizations and institutions, and multinational corporations imposing their power over less developed states. He also justifies the reason for this phenomenon, and the main reason is the advancement in technology in all fields of life. Scholte (2000: 41) merely argues that "contemporary globalization can best be described in one word: deterritorialization, or as the growth of supraterritorial relations among people".

Conceptualization of globalization must not be limited to the understanding of the economic changes that it has brought to the new world system; it must also encompass mono-ecological aspects that it requires, which have a lot of undesired effects, especially for the diverse culture of the Indigenous peoples (Scholte, 2000; Bambas et al., 2000). Such consequences are environmental degradation, inequality among individuals of the society and cultural destruction (Scholte, 2000).

In the era of globalization, where different societies of different populations have gone through social, political and economic development, together with the development of the nation-state system, it has become hard for Indigenous people to adopt a policy of self-sufficiency and independence over their territory as they had in the past (Slowey, 2005). After the end of socialism, a new type of development has emerged, which has certain traits, such as the openness of the borders between nation-states and the free flow of capital and goods, which in turn have paved the way to a globalized economy that is in the hands of transnational corporations owned by those in developed countries (Aylwin, 2006). The effects of globalization on the populations of Indigenous peoples have been met with those peoples' efforts to use globalization as a tool to regain the right to their historical and spiritual ties to their lands.

The self-governance of Indigenous people in a world of globalized economy is the ability of the Indigenous people to participate in the decisions and the regulations that will have a direct effect on them, which should involve their prior consultation to any economic project held in their ancestral territories (Rodríguez-Garavito, 2010). And as Rodolfo Stavenhagen (2003) demonstrates, what the word *territory* holds in its meaning is the concept of culture, religion, spiritual sites, ancestors, the natural environment, water, forests and underground minerals. This basic understanding has clashed with global liberalism, the foundation of transnational bodies like the World Bank and the transnational corporations (TNC), and the abundance of the bilateral agreements between the most powerful economies due to their needs for raw materials and natural resources to strengthen their economies and the developing countries where the Indigenous people reside and are affected by these development projects (Foster, 2012). It is also due to the combination of the spread of neoliberal reforms during the 1980s and the implementation of the Washington Consensus throughout the

1990s (Martinez, 2012). Thus Indigenous peoples' social and cultural existence, as well as their economies, becomes at risk, and a system of governance needs to be developed in order to cope with the emerging world order and the transnationalism that directly affects Indigenous self-identity and ancestral history. These sets of regulations are generated through a process of negotiations among the concerned partners: NGOs, unions, local communities, state entities, corporations (Rodríguez-Garavito, 2010).

Self-Governance of Indigenous Peoples

It is important to consider what the word autonomy or self-governance means in the eye of the Indigenous peoples, and how it is different from how the global economy defines it. It is best portrayed in June Nash's work (2003) when she explains that if we merely translate the word *anatomia* into "just governance," we will be ignoring the cultural perceptions included in the word *autonomy*, such as realizing dignity.

Charles Hale (2005) agreed with Nash when he explained the term *governance*, what it holds for the Indigenous people and why it is contradictory to neoliberalism. He states that *governance* here does not mean the mere claim of a territory people inhabit; rather, it is a demand of a degree of autonomy over the land and the natural resources that contrasts with the concept of "neoliberal multiculturalism." Neoliberal multiculturalism recognizes culture differences as long as they do not inhibit the method of economic development adopted (Hale, 2005).

The long struggle of Indigenous peoples around the world to force the system of nation-states to first consult the population before any development project takes place that affects their land, and thus their wellbeing, has happened to globalization. As Anthony Giddens (2000) says, the spreading out of globalization has led to Indigenous peoples' rights being more visible and vocal around the world; globalization is "the reason for of local cultural identities in different parts of the world" (2000: 31). According to Noam Chomsky, globalization is in the emergence of civil societies who were able to grow and promote their ideologies reaching for many parts of the world, with an aim to see a world that embraces a lot of cultures (2006).

However, Green and Voyageur (1999) see that even if states have agreed to grant justice or to protect some of the rights of the Indigenous people after a very long historical struggle, "it is not out of good will; it is because they want to guarantee safety for present and future investors to create a peaceful investment environment that attracts business and protects the third party interest, the commitment of the colonial state to contemporary justice for Indigenous peoples is linked to its interest in corporate activity, not in justice per se (Green and Voyageur, 1999: 143)."

Agreements do not always serve the best interests of the people. According to Kuokkanen (2006), the treaties and agreements established by the Indigenous people between their governments in most of the cases limited their political and economic autonomy over their territories though some of them granted cultural rights and the right to preserve their identity. I am sure this is a great beginning of raising further demand for rights.

Why is self-governance so important for Indigenous peoples? The importance of autonomy or self-governance or self-determination as a condition for their survival through time for the Indigenous peoples has been a recognized reality (Kuokkanen, 2006). Access to land for production by individuals is a very important aspect of the Indigenous peoples' culture and their understanding of their history—one that is always misunderstood by the non-Indigenous population (Stavenhagen, 2005). For many Indigenous populations the value of the territory is sacred, and it lies in everything that is on and beneath it (Reinsborough, 2002).

The achievement of self-governance for Indigenous peoples is crucial. As Rodolfo Stavenhagen demonstrates, in the world of global economy, economic development and social justice must take place at the same time for effective results on the individuals and the societies and for well-founded economic stability and development (Stavenhagen, 2005). According to Zoomers (2008), "People are attached to their mountains and valleys; local tales and legends reflect the natural environment's importance in daily life. Mountains are mentioned by name, and as people read the landscape in their own way, there are multiple interpretations of local reality" (2008: 973). This in fact speaks about the deep attachment of Andean people to their land and environment. Kuokkanen (2006: 9) explains further the establishment of the Indigenous people that have resulted in this strong connection with their lands, stating that in their understanding the "well-being of the land is the well-being of the human being."

Relocation or compensation for the Indigenous peoples' land and territory is not a practical solution for them because it is like dislocating them not just from their land but from their original identities that they have built throughout history. If such separation occurs, they "will either perish in body or . . . mind and [their] spirits will be altered so that [they] end up mimicking foreign ways" (Burger, 1987: 4).

In fact, the Indigenous peoples are the people who have benefited least from the system of a globalized economy. As Schroeder (2007: 115) elaborates, "the system of global economy has put the demands of the global market ahead of the needs of the local population". Most of the economic outcomes of globalization have led to cultural, environmental and economic damage to their populations. As Cesoratti (2006) contends, the effect of the eco-tourism on their environment, even though it might have helped in raising their income and promoting their culture in the region and throughout the world, has been negative. In order to benefit economically from the neoliberal global system, one must be part of the system. Indigenous peoples have ended up with few economic gains compared to the ecological damages that occur as a result of participating in this system.

The online sales for Indigenous peoples' art brings about the same negative effects on them. Rivers (2005: 2) has raised concerns about its impact, saying that the impact of online sales of Indigenous people's art in the global market can be interpreted as "displaying potential characteristics of culture domination, even exploitation of culture for sheer economic gain." Moreover, Rivers (2005) placed emphasis on the fact that the youth among these Indigenous populations who migrated and left their lands behind in order to achieve short term financial goals ended up losing their culture and identity. The remittances that they send contribute to building the economies of these societies; losing attachment to one's culture can be compensated by the economic development that globalization offers.

Generally, the outcome of the globalized economy did not come out as desired, and it had an instant negative impact and a set of new reforms that John Williamson listed, best known as the Washington consensus, which included some neoliberal reforms of liberalization of trade, liberating foreign direct investment and securing property rights (Williamson and Dalal, 2007). Paul Cooney (2006:1) indicated that during the past two decades "the neoliberal model has dominated economic policies in Latin America and in general, has produced lower wages, an increase in unemployment and poverty for the majority of Latin Americans, as well as financial crises and depressions." Cooney (2006) goes on to present statistics on the statistics of poverty in Latin America before and after these reforms took place. The level of poverty increased by 8 percent in one decade from 1980 to 1990.

After the free trade agreements took place, some economic and development projects began. However, most of the projects of the Indigenous peoples' land and resources excluded them from decision-making. These did not start off with the best terms, and all the Indigenous populations have seen from globalization is the physical, psychological and spiritual damage of their territories and in return their wellbeing (Blaser et al., 2008). As a result of what they have witnessed from the system brought to them by globalization and the harms they have experienced, Indigenous peoples have used it as a tool in creating an alternative system of local governance beside the state (Scholte, 2000). This system of governance is not about seeking power from the state; rather, it is based in the Indigenous peoples' understanding and desire to build an equal world "based on the rotation of representatives," and it stresses the fact that building the community should start from "the bottom up" (Zibechi, 2010: 3).

The marginalization of the Indigenous within the system means that it does not use their knowledge or experience when dealing with the changes these development projects will bring. Moreover, calling their beliefs "myths" because they do not fit into scientific understanding has further marginalized the Indigenous peoples and turned them toward demanding their full collective rights for their territories and everything they represent (Martinez, 2012).

Their misrepresentation continues, even by human rights organizations, which have referred to them as a group of poor, disadvantaged and vulnerable citizens. They need to speak out for themselves and to be the only side allowed to define themselves, their cultures and their histories (Radcliffe et al., 2002). Most of the issues the Indigenous populations face can be summoned in their access to their lands and their resources, and this is still the main problem faced by their communities keeping them discriminated against and marginalized. Their lack of access to proper education and health systems is a very common feature, and another one that is very strong is the inefficiency of the administration of the justice system.

It is said that despite the agreements reached and the peace treaties signed, the human rights violations committed against those Indigenous peoples are always on the rise (Stavenhagen, 2005).

> The struggle of Indigenous peoples for their self determination.
> "We are seeking an explanation for this 'progress' that goes against life. We are demanding that this kind of progress stop. That oil exploration in the heart of the Earth is halted, that the deliberate bleeding of the Earth stops"— Statement of the U'wa people, August 1998.
>
> Statement of the U'wa People, August 8, 1998
> (The Rain Forest Action Network, 2001:2)

Over the past 50 years, the Indigenous peoples have undergone a legal struggle to earn their collective rights back over their territories. It started within their communities and then developed into a regional and international struggle that fit into the globalized legal system of the contemporary world; international bodies have surpassed nation-states' borders and forced them to abide by certain international laws (UNHR, 2013). The movement of transnational activism was formed with a view to protecting the rights of the Indigenous peoples. The UN's Human Rights Commission resolution that addressed a sub-committee to study "the problem of discrimination against Indigenous population and how to eliminate it is considered as an important milestone[1] (Garavito, 2010).

Then a massive movement of the Indigenous peoples, together with some NGOs and scholars and anthropologists, began, which was followed by the formation of an international law institution in 1982 (Garavito, 2010). More than ten years later, in 1994, this working group was able to present the first draft of the Declaration on the Rights of Indigenous Peoples, which after many discussions and meetings led to the final Declaration that was approved by the UN General Assembly in 2007 (Garavito, 2010).

The Draft Declaration on the Rights of Indigenous Peoples states in Article 33: "Indigenous peoples have the right to promote, develop and maintain their institutional structures and their distinctive juridical customs, traditions, procedures and practices, in accordance with internationally recognized human rights standards" (UNGA, 2007). This was an important achievement in the contemporary history of the Indigenous people, which was backed by another important adoption, ILO Convention 169 of 1989 (Rodríguez-Garavito, 2010). These achievements appeared after a long struggle and sacrifice. The concept of the claim of the Indigenous peoples totally contrasted with the neoliberal view of the global economy, in which value only lies in the mere material value of the land and its economic resources.

The International Labour Organization's Convention 169 states in Article 7.1: "The peoples concerned shall have the right to decide their own priorities for the process of development as it affects their lives, beliefs, institutions and spiritual wellbeing and the lands they occupy or otherwise use, and to exercise control, to the extent possible, over their own economic, social and cultural development."

For their Jurisprudence, there is the Inter-American Court of Human Rights. Groups on Indigenous peoples have held yearly sessions with different actors, and they spoke for the social and human rights aspects of the Indigenous people, and the results of their participation usually turned out to be great. Apart from the human rights aspects, Indigenous peoples sought to gain their right of political representation in their countries. This latter goal was achieved in a number of countries, while it is not yet a reality still in other many countries, especially in Asia, Africa and Latin America. In Latin America, for example, the congress in Chile voted against several initiatives that would recognize the Indigenous peoples as peoples who have their complete autonomy over their land and political life. In Africa, even though the Organization of African Unity (OAU) approved the African Charter on Humans and Peoples' Rights, the term *people* was not exactly defined (Stavenhagen, 2005).

The civil organizations formed to advocate for the Indigenous over the years have made great progress and earned recognition from some governments of some states. They have moved from local to regional and then to national and international levels in order to make changes in their life. They were able to be recognized as legitimate partners and participants in the national scene, and they impacted the state policies. Of course, this impact has varied from one country to another, according to certain factors, such as demography, organization skills, and whether the societies surrounding them accept their diversity (Aylwin, 2005).

Martinez (2012) agrees with him and argues that the development of the system of the worldwide transportation and information and communications technologies (ICTs) is one of the main factors that allowed the Indigenous peoples to mobilize beyond their national and local levels. Building a network of sub-regional, regional, national and international networks to ultimately reach their goal in attempt to regain and consolidate their rights was possible because of ICTs.

The Indigenous peoples' struggle to win back at least most of their rights did not come off easily and was characterized by persistence, patience and sacrifices. There was a clash of understanding between the Indigenous peoples' definitions of certain terms—such as belonging, history, a system of governance and self-autonomy over the territory—and what the globalized system sought to implement. These very epistemological differences led the Indigenous peoples around the world to undergo one of the most important battles throughout their history, a battle for their existence against a very powerful, global dominant enemy, which is a world system, in order to preserve their identity and demand collective rights like those they had in the past; they fought to be a part of the system and in the legal framework of the same system that has affected them negatively (Reinsborough, 2002).

A common feature of this long-term fight was the criminalization of the social conflicts of the Indigenous peoples—on the Western side—and the defamation of their reputation by saying that it is against the national interest or against the ethics and morals of the state and the society (Martinez, 2012). Throughout their journey of calling for autonomy over their land, they found themselves facing the "racist and stereotypical representation of the Native as backwards and primitive" (Martinez, 2012: 115).

And as noted by Rodolfo Stavenhagen (2005), the conflict over land and resources negatively affected the Indigenous population because of the lack of a legal framework that would state these peoples' rights over their lands, and this has led to the migration of some of Indians to other parts of Mexico and Central America, which threatens their wellbeing and the survival of their culture. Earlier, on a different occasion, Rodolfo Stavenhagen pointed out the issues that the Indigenous peoples suffer from as a result of the globalized economy:

> In various United Nations and other forums, Indigenous organizations have signaled their concern about negative impacts of major development projects on their environments, livelihoods, lifestyles and survival. One of the recurrent issues is the loss of land and territories that Indigenous communities suffer. The lack of control over their natural resources has become a widespread worry. Very often these projects entail involuntary displacements and resettlement of Indigenous communities which happen to lie in the way of a dam, an airport, a game reserve, a tourist resort, a mining operation, a pipeline, a major highway, etc. As a result, violations of civil and political, economic, social and cultural rights occur with increasing frequency, prompting Indigenous peoples to launch major protests or resistance campaigns in order to bring public attention to their plight, besides engaging the judicial system or appealing for administrative redress, as well as lobbying the political system (United Nations (Commission on Human Rights, 2003: Par. 19).

It is only through resistance that Indigenous peoples won a degree of recognition and a right to remain distinct from the ideologies that their governments represent. According to Martinez, what is more important than including all the rights of Indigenous peoples in the domestic laws and the international agreements is to make sure that these governments abide by them. This implies that their struggle should continue until governments are faced with constant pressure from the people, NGOs, international and regional institutions such as the UN, ILO and OAS.

The U'wa People from Columbia and West Venezuela

U'wa people are a group of more than 8,000 Indigenous people residing in the northeast of Columbia (Mander and Tauli-Corpuz, 2003; Niezen, 2003; Rodríguez-Garavito and Arenas, 2005). They have no written language and their culture and language are preserved through songs. Their existence during all these centuries was through older generations' teachings on how to preserve the land they reside on and make use of their resources without doing any harm to Mother Nature. It is in their ancestral history that they consider themselves as the sole guardians of the forests and the species living on them, plants and animals. They have managed to survive a long time, and many people have been surprised by the U'wa people's ability to preserve their lands and resources for centuries; they even survived the Spanish conquistadors. Now, Columbia is a country exhausted by the civil war with the rebels, and the government needs to increase their foreign reserves by putting their hands on the natural resources that are lying under the territories of the U'wa. Their religion demands they keep the harmony between the layers of creation; earth, water, oil, mountain and sky; the autonomy over their ancestral lands is essential and important because they are following their religion (Rodríguez-Garavito and Arenas, 2005).

Now the U'wa are fighting transnational corporations (TNC) and the country's new economy, which think that the U'wa are preventing the economy of the country of 40 million people from flourishing. Moreover, the oil industry on their land are attracting conflicts between the armed guerrillas and the Columbian government, thus destroying the environment of the U'wa people and threatening their existence (Ulloa, 2003: 52). The U'wa people tried to explain to the government the value of their ancestral territories in their culture and the environmental damage that might occur if the drilling of oil took place, and yet the government agreed to grant permission to the Occidental Petroleum Corporation (Oxy) to work on the U'wa territories.

The U'wa people first turned to the Constitutional Court of Columbia in order to defend their property rights and demand the cessation of the drilling. They based their claims on an old warrant given to the Tuneba Nation from the Spanish Crown that entitled them to have full access and control over the ancestral land soil and subsoil. The Court ruled in their favor, summoning the ILO Convention N.169 and the 1991 constitution. However, this decision was overthrown by the Council of the State of Columbia, who stated that they had previously notified the population about the drilling and they have no further obligation towards the people. So the U'wa people had to turn to other peaceful ways of denouncing what is happening on their territory. First they organized massive rallies, general peasants' strikes, road blockades, and hunger strikes by the Indigenous members of the Columbia Congress during the time of legislation; their most powerful and strong way of showing their anger was their pact of committing massive suicide if the drilling did not stop by jumping off the cliff (Niezen, 2003; Rodríguez-Garavito and Arenas, 2005; Barker, 2007; Ulloa, 2003). One of their tribal leaders, who had a very important role in the international campaign to stop the exploitation of oil on their territories, said in a speech (Martinez, 2012): "We would rather die, protecting everything that we hold sacred, than lose everything that makes us U'wa" (Ulloa, 2003: 47).

The movement was able to go global and their supporters started a negative marketing campaign on the Oxy headquarters in Los Anglos (Martinez, 2012). Finally, in 2002, the Oxy was forced to leave the territories of U'wa. However, the following year, in 2003, Ecopetrol, which is a company owned by the Columbian state, is now drilling over their land. The government is trying to establish a policy of intercultural dialogue with the U'wa people, who still refuse the drilling that is taking place on their land. They have gone to the Inter-American Court. Ecopetrol has chosen not to explore in the reserve until today.

One of the main demonstrations of triumph throughout the history of the Indigenous peoples' struggle for their survival was the election of the president

Evo Morales, an Aymara, of Bolivia in 2005, as the first Indigenous president in its history. Bolivia is a state where the majority of its population is Indigenous (Cesarotti, 2000). Recently, the Indigenous peoples in Latin America have led movements that managed to earn some of their lawful claims in their countries— for example, their political representation and participation and the recognition of their right to the complete autonomy over their historical territories and their resources (Aylwin, 2005).

Latin American countries gave legal recognition to some of the Indigenous peoples' rights within their national constitutions, as in these cases: "Panama (1971), Nicaragua (1986), Brazil (1988), Colombia (1991), México (1992 y 2001), Guatemala (1985), Paraguay (1992), Peru (1993), Argentina (1994), Bolivia (1994), Ecuador (1994 and 1998) and Venezuela (1999) have reformed their constitutions to give some kind of recognition to Indigenous peoples (or people)" (Aylwin, 2005: 13). However, in all Latin American countries the right of control of the subsoil land still is not granted to the Indigenous peoples and is still an exclusive right of the nation-states (Aylwin, 2005).

Indigenous Populations in Mexico

The Indigenous peoples constitute 14 percent of the 13 million population in Mexico—the largest Indigenous population in Latin America (Deruyttere, 2001). Part of this population is called the Zapatista—a leading Indigenous resistance movement located in the southern Mexico—and it is one of the most successful movements, gaining worldwide solidarity (Cesarotti, 2000). Like many other Indigenous movements, the Zapatista emerged from the economic, environmental and cultural damage of globalization. Their campaigns were really successful in driving the international capitalist system off their natural and local resources (Collier and Collier, 2005: 457). The Zapatista use globalization to reach out for the outside world, and they say that they have used "the very processes of globalization that they have challenged"; "some call the rebellion the first 'postmodern' revolution due to its use of the media and internet" (Collier and Collier, 2005: 451).

Mander and Tauli-Corpuz (2006) says, "it's clear that the forces that at first exploited the Indigenous peoples in Bolivia have ultimately provided them with greater voice and respect." Then he goes on, explaining the wide-ranging consequences of popular demonstration: "They are joining with networks . . . to raise their voices against free trade pacts on the international arena. And they are doing this within a context of expanded struggles for ethnic recognition, autonomy and self-government" (Mander and Tauli-Corpuz, 2006: 182).

The Indigenous peoples of Chiapas, who are coffee producers, were pushed into poverty because of the free trade policies in the region. As a result, they have created their own economic program of organic production and were supported by the Zapatistas and the solidarity movements and organizations (Tavanti, 2003: 2). The Zapatistas have created an Alternative Economy Program, which includes programs like e-trade and fair trade. The program has included the Indigenous women making some handmade traditional clothing at home to sell to the buyer directly with the help of this program (Smith and Kroondyk, 2009). These programs have been created to defy one of the most important free trade agreements that took place last century between Canada, United States and Mexico: the North American Free Trade Agreement (NAFTA). Most of the outcomes of this agreement have directly affected the Indigenous peoples living in the southern part of Mexico (Villarreal and Fergusson, 2015) because the agreements made it easy to buy a free spot of lands to be owned by landless peasants, as a result this opened a door for privatization and the land and taking control over the size of production.

Note

1. (ECOSOC), Res. 1589(L) 7, U.N. Doc. E/5044 (1971).

5 Improving Health by Self-Governance

Indigenous struggles have long been against injustices perpetrated not only by colonial rulers but also by modern states. The injustices primarily are the displacement from the land or denial of access to the land to enjoy their own cultural mores. In addition, for centuries, Indigenous peoples around the world have been struggling to establish the right to govern their nations and their lands. For most of that time, colonial powers denied them that right—a right today we call Aboriginal self-government (Penikett, 2012a). Britain fought a second war against Indigenous allies of the French who were led by Pontiac, a Ottawa warrior chief, after the British and Iroquois armies defeated the French in 1759. That resulted in the Royal Proclamation of 1763, which recognized First Nation governments as original landowners. Eventually, the Proclamation would lead to the negotiation of almost 400 Indian treaties in the United States and Canada. In 1876 Parliament passed the Indian Act, which turned the treaty signatories into dependents of the federal state. However, Canada's Aboriginal peoples did not give up their struggle for land and governance rights (Penikett, 2012b).

Penikett (2012b) offers six definitions of self-governance: firstly, by definition, Aboriginal government is something that colonial authorities sought to deny First Nations. The second one is that "self-government describes the right of a First Nation to govern itself, make decisions for its future and exercise a full range of jurisdiction and authority over its lands, peoples and resources (Micha, 2012: 3)". "A third definition might state that Aboriginal self-government in Canada can encompass both local or municipal and province-like powers" (Penikett, 2012b: 4). The fourth one affirms that Aboriginal self-government is about enjoying law-making powers as well as the administration and enforcement of those laws. The fifth definition is about gaining collective title to a large tracts and managing those lands and the communities on them. And the last of form of Aboriginal self-governance is about negotiating accommodation agreements, co-management, co-jurisdiction, resource-revenue, and other intergovernmental arrangements to empower itself and reasserting legitimate authority over its people, lands, and resources (Penikett, 2012).

Alfred (2009: 41) pointed out an important aspect to colonialism: "the colonially-generated cultural disruption affecting First Nations . . . compounds the effects of dispossession to create near total psychological, physical and financial dependency on the state." This kind of dependency has been a crisis primarily because of the complex living of the Indigenous with social suffering, historical trauma and cultural dislocation. In such circumstances, opportunities for self-sufficient, healthy and autonomous lives for them have shrunk. Alfred further argues that racism, expropriation of lands, extinguishment of rights, wardship, and welfare dependency are important constituents of colonial characters, and it is the reality for the Indigenous lives and more so for the women and children.

Self-government is viewed by most Indigenous peoples as a way to [re]gain control over the management of matters that directly affect them and to preserve their cultural identities. Self-government is referred to as an inherent right, a pre-existing right rooted in Indigenous peoples' long occupation and government of the land before European settlement. Many Indigenous peoples speak of sovereignty and self-government as responsibilities given to them by the Creator and of a spiritual connection to the land. They do not seek to be granted self-government by governments, but rather to have citizens recognize that Indigenous governments existed long before the arrival of Europeans and to establish the conditions that would permit the revival of their governments.

The right to self-determination can serve as a perpetuation of their cultural practices. Self-determination enables an Indigenous population to thrive in its culture and thus develop a sustainable economy. This is how they can enjoy their traditions and basic human rights. There is no doubt that Indigenous communities are threatened by extinction, and their members are among the poorest and most marginalized members of our societies (Zardo, 2013). The belief is that if there are inclusive policies, Indigenous communities would gradually assimilate to the larger societies and cultures.

Indigenous peoples' right to self-determination was granted and approved in 2007 by the UN General Assembly. This allows them political status to pursue their economic, social and cultural development. "The interplay between the right to self-determination, the collective right to culture, and the individual rights of members of the community is what lends significant complexity to the issue of how human rights law should deal with gender discrimination within Indigenous communities" (Zardo, 2013: 1060). Individual rights as well as collective rights are primary components of protection of minorities from discrimination by the majorities.

With the historical relations of Indigenous peoples to their land and territory as the material base of their survival, they have an inherent right to their land. Because of the historical injustices committed against Indigenous peoples—disregarding their interests, welfare and human rights and their collective right to exist—Indigenous peoples need to be protected to ensure their continuing survival. Without the material base of their existence, Indigenous peoples cannot practice their own distinct cultures and ways of life.

Indigenous peoples have begun to claim their right to self-determination, which is their collective right practiced in nation-states as their right to development. This collective right guarantees them the right to pursue their development in accordance with their own culture and ways of life. It is widely believed that health care professionals have significant role in promoting Indigenous health. This can happen daily for those caring for patients of all ages in a wide variety of settings, including rural communities, urban environments, or tertiary care centers. Advocacy in key areas plays important role in promoting Indigenous health. These include helping researchers, policy makers and health care providers to understand the history of Indigenous peoples, with the negative legacy of colonization; the role of the social determinants of health; and the urgent need for increased education and employment (Macaulay, 2009). It also important that we advocate for more Indigenous health care professionals; multidisciplinary teams; increased Indigenous self-government, with control of programs including health and education; improved care for patients, families, and communities through adequate funding and relevant programs that are developed with Indigenous input and are appropriately evaluated; and research directed by or undertaken in partnership with Indigenous peoples.

Health and Self-Governance Correlates

A growing aging population in a particular country results in increased dependence on welfare system, especially health services. The interplay of health of the aging population and Indigenous peoples has crucial implications for policy makers and researchers. Indigenous people have a lower median age, meaning that the aging population among the Indigenous is lower than it is among non-Indigenous peoples. This might be one of the reasons why researchers have paid less attention to this group (Beatty and Berdahl, 2011). However, currently the growth is faster than the non-Indigenous. As a result, these seniors become a neglected section of the society. Indigenous seniors suffer poorer health than non-Indigenous seniors. There is no doubt that aborigines lack socioeconomic supports.

The idea that integrating the Indigenous population into the mainstream population would be helpful to address their needs has been proven wrong in the sense that this initiative may threaten their cultural life. For example, Stanton (2011) observes that as one step of such an initiative, the government of Canada intended to integrate Indigenous children into the non-Indigenous culture. In doing so, the government required them to attend church-run schools (International Symposium on the Social Determinants of Indigenous Health, 2007).

The determinants of Indigenous health are different from those of the mainstream population (Czyzewski, 2011). Partly, this is how Indigenous populations perceive health compared to Western biomedical definitions. Some of the previously cited mechanisms are actually identified as distal determinants. That an Indigenous SDH framework should be different from the conventional framework emphasized that the latter's indicators were not reliable for all (International Symposium on the Social Determinants of Indigenous Health, 2007).

Colonialism has had direct impact on health of the Indigenous populations. To quote again Czyzewski (2011: 6) "Colonialism is the guiding force that manipulated the historic, political, social, and economic contexts shaping Indigenous/ state/non-Indigenous relations and acounts for the public erasure of political and economic marginalization, and racism today. These combined components shape the health of Indigenous peoples." This in fact endorses what I mentioned about the impact of colonialism on Indigenous health.

Many researchers confirmed that colonization and social determinants have crucial impacts on Aboriginal people's health (Reading and Wien, 2009; Russell and de Leeuw, 2012). The effect of colonization on the Indigenous population is evident from the specific case of the British colonization of the Australian continent. The British did not recognize Indigenous rights to the land. Loss of land forced them to leave for small inland areas where food was scarce. The introduction of diseases such as smallpox and measles, against which the Aborigines had no immunity as they had never been exposed to them before, caused many aborigines to die without treatment. Family ties were severed because the Europeans took Indigenous children out of their families to schools where other European children studied. There have been deliberate actions to destroy Indigenous culture.

In Taiwan, for example, there are about 513,000 Aboriginal inhabitants who may have occupied the island about 8,000 years before the Han majority arrived on the island (Blust, 1999, cited in Lee and Chen, 2014). Taiwan has undergone various colonial periods. Indigenous populations were labeled and categorized in those periods as mountain tribes and wild aborigines etc. Launched in 1984, The Taiwan Aboriginal People's Movement (TAPM) sent a representative to the United Nations Working Group on Indigenous Populations in 1988 when they began advocacy with the government to have policies revised to better address their causes (Lee and Chen, 2014). As a result, the Taiwanese government recognized the legal status of its Indigenous groups in 1994, and they were renamed the "earliest inhabitants."

The burden of diseases is as disproportionately distributed, meaning that Indigenous peoples carry a higher burden of diseases compared with non-Indigenous peoples. The disparities remaining in health between Indigenous and non-Indigenous populations of many countries is alarming (Wong et al., 2014). It is not just in developing or underdeveloped countries. It is prevalent within developed countries as well. What is striking is that even in developed countries, in Australia, for instance, infant mortality among Indigenous people is three times higher than that of the non-Indigenous population (Wong et al., 2014).

It is important that we touch upon universal health coverage, which was proposed as an answer to the existing challenges to accessing to health care systems to ensure that health care is affordable and available to all people. "Universal health coverage relies on a strong, efficient, and well-run health system that meets priority needs through people-centered, integrated care: One that is affordable, provides access to essential medicines and technology, and has sufficient capacity of well trained motivated health workers" (WHO, 2012: 11).

One of the significant challenges in improving universal health coverage is finances. However, appropriate infrastructure, qualified and culturally sensitive personnel, supportive socioeconomic and policy environments, and adequate implementing structures are also important determinants of universal health coverage (Wong et al., 2014).

Many countries in Asia, especially in South East Asia, have been providing better health services than many other countries. However, a huge number of hill tribe households in Thailand and Myanmar, for instance, were not accorded citizenship status. Thus they were denied access to state health systems (Hu, 2009). In Malaysia, Indigenous peoples (or Orang Asli) are classified into three main groups and sub-divided further into 18 ethnic sub-groups (Department of Aboriginal Development, 2012). The Orang Asli are the oldest population group recorded to inhabit the Peninsula.

Colonization has had impacts on many aspects of the Indigenous life. According to Baskin (2007), colonization is the determinant of Aboriginal health. Residential schools in Canada or in Scandinavian countries and elsewhere for Indigenous children have been presented as examples by many as colonialism (Reading and Wien, 2009; Juutilainen et al., 2014). These schools in fact produce racialism as well as social, political, and economic inequalities. In the long run, these inequalities affect determinants of health.

"The main goal of the residential schools, whether it was written into policy or implied by institutional practices, was to assimilate Indigenous children into the dominant culture. Indigenous children were taught that their own language and cultural practices were inferior to the dominant culture and were instilled with the notion that they were 'less than' the majority society" (Juutilainen et al., 2014: 3). Aboriginal children constitute about six percent of the Canadian child population in 2006 (Statistics Canada, 2009). There are about 132 schools supported by the federal government in Canada, and operated 'jointly' with Anglican, Catholic, and Presbyterian churches. There are widespread complaints that children have been forcibly removed from their homes and often taken far from their communities. Some of these children have died while attending residential schools (Aboriginal Affairs and Northern Development Canada, 2008).

Governments in many countries have played strategies to integrate and assimilate children into the 'mainstream.' Residential school is one such strategy, although these strategies are not in place as a written policy. In Finland, Saami language and culture were repressed by teaching in boarding schools only in Finnish. Saami children were forbidden to speak their mother tongue at school and in the dormitories. Thus Sami culture was hindered and many of them lost their language.

Prior to colonization, Aboriginal child care was different from that in other populations, which means that they would care for their children in line with their own cultural norms and practices. "The existence and continuity of customary care traditions in Canada have been documented in a number of court cases" (Zlotkin, 2009 cited in Sinha and Kozlowski, 2013: 5). For instance, grandparents are considered the primary caregivers of children in First Nations communities. Tactics used in assimilating aborigines into mainstream were many. In health services, since the beginning of the contact with the Aboriginal people, non-Aboriginal physicians used European style practices of health services in order to promote the assimilation of Aboriginal Peoples (Kelm, 1998). Cultural sensitivity of the aborigines were not taken into consideration while asking about health issues by the family medicine practitioners.

Even with the growing recognition of Indigenous peoples' rights, these rights are still being violated with impunity in most countries with Indigenous peoples among their population. Thus, more and more Indigenous peoples are now putting up stronger resistance, and forging solidarity relations, as well as intensifying their local struggles in defense of their land and their very survival (Mackay, 2002).

Latin America: Latin America has witnessed considerable development in the battle for gaining self-government. The political influence of Indigenous people in Latin America, measured by Indigenous political parties, Indigenous elected representatives, constitutional provisions for Indigenous people or Indigenous-tailored health and education policies has grown in the last 15 years (Hall and Patrinos, 2004). In the last 20 years, voters in Bolivia, Guatemala and elsewhere have significantly increased. Indigenous people and Indigenous political parties have also won municipal and mayoral elections across Latin America (Mackay, 2002).

The Indigenous movement, for example, in Guatemala is both the consequence of a long history of oppression and injustices, and the result of a worldwide mobilization trend initiated by Indigenous peoples of developed and democratic countries in order to obtain political recognition. During the Spanish conquest and colonial period, legal institutions oppressed Indigenous people by forcing them to work and give away their lands (Postero, 2000). An estimated 75 million Indigenous people died in the sixteenth and seventeenth centuries in Latin America due to forced labor, wars and epidemics under Spanish colonialism (IPS, 1999; Crowshoe, 2005). The majority of the Bolivian people are of Indigenous origin. Bolivia has one of the highest poverty levels in Latin America, with 63 percent of the population living in conditions of extreme poverty. Sixty percent of the population has no access to drinking water. The situation is most critical in the rural areas, where 94 percent of homes do not have access to basic services. Some 78 percent of poverty-stricken rural homes do not have access to drinking water and 72 percent lack sanitary services. Various regions suffer from endemic illnesses associated with poverty. Malaria, tuberculosis and *chagas* disease, combined with diarrhea and respiratory infections, cause a high prevalence of infant mortality (Gaviria and Raphael, 2001). The wave of Indigenous claims in Latin America, which started in the late 1980s, is part of a broader international trend in favor of the minorities' rights, especially for Indigenous Peoples of North America (Peeler, 2000).

Given that Indigenous peoples' struggles to empower themselves "are occurring in a global political space in which claims to authenticity are a critical dimension of legitimacy" (Brosius, 1999: 181), it is often the case that Indigenous peoples and their supporters have to resort to the same set of dominant images of Indigenousness that states, interest groups, advocates and experts use to advance their own agendas. In Paraguay, for example, non-Indigenous supporters promote the rights of Indigenous peoples, including rights to land and specific forms of development, by using a definition of Indigenousness that includes traits such as harmonious relations with nature and generosity with neighbors (Peeler, 2000).

Abuses and exploitation by the colonial empires for centuries lead the Indigenous in Latin America in struggle of political recognition. The wave of constitutional reforms incorporating Indigenous claims started with Nicaragua in 1987 and it continued with Brazil in 1988 and so on (Mendoza, 2002). Indigenous movements nowadays have been shaping public policies of many countries in the world. In Latin America alone, between 1987 and 1999, eleven countries enacted constitutional reforms, which included recognition of Indigenous people culture and their rights (Mendoza, 2002). However, although most of the States in Latin America have made constitutional changes to recognize Indigenous rights, the balance of the last few decades is critical, with evidence of rules being either ineffective or breached (United Nations, 2006).

Colombia and Venezuela have included specific mechanisms for Indigenous political representation in their respective contributions. Now Colombia's contribution guarantees two Indigenous representatives in the senate of 100 members, while it is only three for Venezuela (Agrawal et al., 2012). While around half of the total population in Guatemala (49 percent) is Indigenous, less than half of them are registered to vote. Although there is a presence of representation at the local level, at the national level, presence is minimal at the executive branch, in the congress and in the judiciary (Mendoza, 2002). Bolivia has a population of 8.4 million inhabitants, with 60 percent living in rural areas, and the majority of them are of Indigenous origin. Indigenous peoples in Bolivia are the most affected in Latin America as 63 percent of the population live in extreme poverty (Gaviria and Raphael 2001).

North America: Indigenous self-government has become a prominent issue worldwide, especially in the countries in North America over the past several decades. While attention focused on constitutional reform between 1980s and early 1990s, the agenda has shifted toward policy and legislative changes in recent years. Significant developments in 1998–99 included the federal government response to the Report of the Royal Commission on Aboriginal Peoples (RCAP) in January 1998, the conclusion of the Nisga'a Final Agreement in August 1998, and establishment of Nunavut in April 1999. Aboriginal peoples in Canada are defined in the Constitution Act, 1982 as Indians, Inuit and Métis (Wherrett, 1999).

It is worth looking at the Alberta Métis Settlements Accords and agreements[1] of the late 1980s and Nunavut.[2] Although there are differences between these two contemporary forms of self-government the similarities between them are striking. Both sets of negotiation with government began in the mid-1970s and ended in the early 1990s. The new governance structures of the Settlements and the Nunavut government are circumscribed by more than one piece of legislation. One major difference between these two forms of Aboriginal self-government is that the Alberta Métis Settlements Councils are clear examples of ethnic governments that are elected and operated by members of a particular ethnic group. Nunavut is an example of a public government in which anyone who meets residence requirements, regardless of ethnicity, can participate in the election of the government (Wall, 1998).

Critics of current forms of Indigenous self-government in Canada view them as little more than convenient arrangements that allow Aboriginal people administrative responsibility for services which are ultimately controlled by the federal or provincial government (Dacks, 1986). Self-government proposals also have their critics among the very people for whom it is intended. For example, Inuit women have objected to many parts of the Nunavut agreement mainly because of concerns about an emphasis on conventional southern Canadian notions of resource management. They also had concerns and about an emphasis on the economic, social and political roles and issues for men at the expense of those of women in Nunavut (Inuit Women's Association, 1993).

Oceania: As the numbers of Indigenous peoples began slowly to increase, an Aboriginal Advancement (i.e. civil rights) movement in Australia developed with the aims to give Indigenous peoples, including Torres Strait Islanders, the full rights and entitlements of citizenship (United Nations, 2006). Until the late 1950s and early 1960s, the various states denied them these rights. In 1967 the country voted to amend the constitution to give the federal government jurisdiction over policies regarding Indigenous people, and in 1973 the government established the Department of Aboriginal Affairs in Australia. This agency sponsored or promoted programs in housing, education, health, land ownership, business, and legal and administrative reform. In 1991 the department was succeeded by the Aboriginal and Torres Strait Islander Commission (ATSIC) and spent $900 million annually to support the principle of Indigenous self-determination (Inuit Women's Association, 1993).

The search for better work, education, and health care opportunities, along with the mechanization of farming and herding operations that formerly required the Aborigines' labor, has prompted many Aborigines to move to major cities. The collapse of the pearling industry, which formerly employed many Torres Strait Islanders, has caused many of these people to move to the mainland. As the Aboriginal political movement has gained in strength, it has aimed at winning back for particular communities the lands their ancestors once owned. As a result, by 1991 a seventh of Australia's land area had come under Indigenous ownership. In 1992 the High Court of Australia ruled in favor of a group claiming recognition of their rights of customary ownership of land on Murray Island in Torres Strait. The ruling in this so-called Mabo cause (named after Eddie Mabo, a plaintiff) overturned the legal assumption that Australia had been terra nullius (unowned land) before its occupation by Europeans (Tebtebba, 2004). With regional differences, the health status of Indigenous Australians is poor. The relative mortality gap between Indigenous and non-Indigenous people appears to have widened in recent years (Kunitz, 2000). Aboriginal and Torres Strait Islander people bear a much greater burden of poor health than other Australians, beginning early in life and continuing throughout their life cycle.

As discussed earlier, globalization does not have equal impact on all regions and communities. The public health risks that have acquired global significance are associated with infectious diseases, occupational hazards and transboundary pollution. These are the legal and institutional responses of states and international organizations; the role of non-state actors in global health governance from the mid-nineteenth century until the mid-twentieth century; the effectiveness of the global health governance regimes constructed in this period; and the lessons of the first century of international health diplomacy for people currently struggling with global risks to public health and the politics they generate (Fidler, 2001).

In New Zealand, Maori, who are full and equal citizens of New Zealand, have been represented in Parliament since the nineteenth century with four seats reserved for them. They later became members of Parliament on the general list as representatives of the various political parties. Currently, Parliament has 21 Maori members of Parliament (about 17.3 percent of the total seats) (ILO, 2007). Fifty-five percent of declared Maori voters are currently on the Maori roll. A recent development is the emergence of the Maori Party, which at its first poll in September 2005 won four seats in Parliament. In the current Government, there are six ministers of Maori descent. The MMP system,[3] whatever its limitations, has broadened democracy in New Zealand and should continue governing the electoral process in the country to ensure a solid Maori voice in Parliament and guarantee democratic pluralism (United Nations, 2006). Whereas *iwi* and *hapu* (tribes and sub-tribes) are acknowledged traditional units of Maori social organization with whom the Government is settling Treaty claims, they have no formally recognized governance powers. In relation to historical Treaty settlements, the Government's policy is to settle with large natural groups that include *iwi, hapu* and *whanau* (families) (Wall, 1998).[4]

The law of the land prohibits discrimination against Indigenous peoples; however, there was a continuing pattern of disproportionate numbers of Maori on unemployment and welfare rolls, in prison, among school dropouts, in infant mortality statistics, and among single-parent households (Tebtebba, 2004). The government created the position of Coordinating Minister for Race Relations review all government policies and programs to ensure that they were directed at persons in need, without racial bias. Government policy recognized a special role for Indigenous people and their traditional values and customs, including cultural and environmental issues that affected commercial development. The Ministry of Maori Development, in cooperation with several Maori NGOs, sought to improve the status of Indigenous people (United Nations, 2006).

Asia: About half of the 200 million of Asia's Indigenous peoples live in India. I am highlighting here the case of Indigenous self-government in Bangladesh. Historically, Indigenous peoples have been known to be living in the Chittagong Hill Tracts (CHT) for centuries, with their own forms of governance and sociopolitical institutions. Today, there are about 600,000 Indigenous peoples in the CHT, out of a total population of approximately a million (974,445) (Census, 1991; Dictaan-Bang-oa, 2004). The Chittagong Hill Tracts (CHT) peace accord was signed in 1997 between the government and the Parbatya Chattagram Jana Sanghati Samity (PCJSS). Under the framework of the constitution of Bangladesh and having fullest and firm confidence in the sovereignty and integrity of Bangladesh, the national Committee on CHT Affairs, on behalf of the government of the People's Republic of Bangladesh and the PCJSS, on behalf of the inhabitants of the Chittagong Hill Tracts, with an objective to elevate political, social, cultural, educational and financial autonomy and to expedite socioeconomic development process of all citizens in CHT, arrived at the agreement (Ramasubramanian, 2005).

Self-Government System for the Indigenous in Bangladesh

In order to get rid of longstanding deprivation, the Indigenous people organized themselves and demanded regional autonomy. During the British India period, CHT had the special status of an autonomously administered district. The Government of India Act of 1935 declared CHT as a "Totally Excluded Area." Under such arrangement, CHT people enjoyed relative autonomy under traditional tribal chiefs, which was administered by the central government (Dictaan-Bang-oa, 2004). After the partition of British India in 1947, CHT came under Pakistan. They lost its special status and autonomy under an amendment to the *Pakistani Constitution* in 1963. The amendment eliminated immigration restrictions and allowed migration of large scale Bengali Settlers into CHT, by whom land and resources of the Jumma people were abused and misappropriated.

The conflict of CHT was intensified greatly when the Government of Pakistan built the Kaptai Hydro-Electric Dam in 1962. The project inundated 54,000 acres—nearly 40 percent—of the most excellent agricultural land, and relocated about 100,000 Indigenous people, mostly the Chakmas. Ninety miles of roads and 10 square miles of reserved forest were also inundated by the project (Ramasubramanian, 2005). The impact of this dam was so influential that a whole generation had to suffer. Thus the *paharis* (inhabitants of the hill) used to call it a Kaptai 'death trap' (Chakraborty, 2004). Chakraborty (2004) in her study found that people still recognize those upsetting memories caused by the building of the dam. She concludes that the feelings of people in CHT who grew up in that time still remain fresh, and they consider the dam a chronicle of losing home. That was a point of departure for thousands of CHT people, whose lives did not return to the same.

Another factor that contributed to the development of CHT conflict was the identity crisis of the Hill people. The Hill people were alienated from the mainstream society through a series of social-political manipulations, which started with the British and continued through the post Bangladesh period, in view of creating 'otherness' (politically, culturally, and socially). Their crisis of identity started in 1947 when they were placed under Pakistan despite strongly appealing to be merged with India since most of them were non-Muslim. The demand of Hill people to merge with India caused them to be accused of being pro-Indian (Mohsin, 2000). However, their demands were not entertained by the post independence rulers of Bangladesh. After the independence of Bangladesh, their demands were also rejected by the then Prime Minister Sheikh Mujibur Rahsman; instead, they were advised to assimilate to the new, nationalist Bengali Identity (Aminuzzaman and Kabir, 2005).

Such definition of nationalism was refused by the Hill people under the leadership of Manobendra Narayan Larma, who raised their disagreement in the parliament by saying that: "You cannot impose your national identity on others. I am Chakma not a Bengali. I am a citizen of Bangladesh, Bangladeshi. You are also a Bangladeshi but your national identity is Bengali . . . They (Hill people) can never become Bengali." However, their disagreement did not make any mark on the Bengali policy makers, who saw Bengali nationalism as all encircling. But the Hill people did not accept such nationalism, which excluded their cultural identities. Thus they were demanding a constitutional guarantee that would safeguard their rights, privileges and cultural uniqueness. Continued refusal of the government of Bangladesh to recognize their cultural uniqueness gave birth to the discontent among Hill people, which contributed to the development of Parbatya Chattagram Jana Samhati Samiti (PCJSS) on 7 March 1972 under the leadership of Manobendra Narayan Larma, through which grievances of the Hill people could be raised.

The root of the CHT's crisis lies in the policies of the government of Bangladesh, which seeks to establish a homogenous Bangali Muslim society by destroying the ethnic identity of the Indigenous Jumma people. About 500,000 illegal plains settlers were implanted into the CHT during 1979–1983 by providing inducements. The Bangali Muslim population, only around 2 percent of the total population of the CHT in 1947, has swung to as high as 49 percent today; the Jumma population, in 1941 constituting 98 percent of the total population, has dwindled to as low as 51 percent (in 2003). If sustained Islamization policies continue, the Jumma people may soon become a minority in their own homeland.

Another contributor to the development of CHT conflict was the initiatives of the successive governments of Bangladesh to solve an inherently political and ethnic problem through military solutions. The problem was initially dealt with through economic development programs, and as a response, the then government formed the CHT Development Board in 1976. Yet these development programs were run by the military and geared towards reinforcing its power in the area; the programs thus amplified prejudice, annoyed the CHT people and increased their penury (Roy, 2000). It is claimed that Bengali settlers, with the help of the army, very often grabbed lands of the Hill people.

The army's ongoing presence has also resulted in serious human rights violations. On 23 August 2004, Rinku Chakma, a UPDF supporter, was killed in military custody in Matiranga of Khagrachari district, after being subjected to serious torture at the Matiranga bazaar in full public view. On 6 August 2004, five members of UPDF were arrested under false accusations (No. G.R. 167/04) at Khagrachari police station. Mithun Chakma and Rupan Chakma, president and vice president of the Hill Students Council respectively, and Ms. Sonali Chakma, president of the Hill Watch Human Rights Forum, were brutally beaten with firewood. The arrest and torture of ordinary Jummas are commonplace occurrences, as reported by the Asian Center for Human Rights (ACHR, 2004).

Demand for Autonomy: After Bangladesh's independence, the Parbatya Chattagram Jana Samhati Samiti (hereinafter PCJSS) was formed in 1972, with the aim of achieving regional autonomy for CHT Indigenous people according to how they themselves envisioned it. The Shanti Bahini (Peace Brigade) was formed as the armed wing of the PCJSS in 1973, with the intention of defending against terrorist attack, rape, torture and looting by Bangali settlers and armed forces (Sing, 1996. 132). On the other hand, the United Peoples Democratic Front (hereinafter

UPDF) was formed on 26 December 1998, opposing the Chittagong Hill Tracts
Accord, 1997, because it failed to address fundamental demands of Jumma people
(as it was argued by the groups of people who established UPDF). UPDF was
committed to establish right of self-determination through full autonomy for the
Indigenous people in CHT (Roy, 2000).

These two Jumma groups remained busy in opposing others for the last ten
years. Moreover, several smaller Indigenous groups feel unrepresented and thus
dislike the fact that Shanti Bahini (the political wing of the Indigenous guerrilla
movement) is in charge of implementing the peace agreement. Fratricidal kill-
ings between two Jumma political parties, the PCJSS and the UPDF, have not
helped the situation, either. Rather, the existence of common Jummas is more
difficult because of the killing, maiming and kidnapping of hundreds of Jumma.
These crimes have been perpetrated by both parties. The refusal of the PCJSS—
its aim is to claim itself sole representative of the Jummas—to even dialogue
with the UPDF has excluded all possibilities for peace. This is despite the fact
that both UPDF activists and JSS cadres have been victims of atrocities by the
Bangladeshi security forces. Ordinary Jummas are thus left to defend themselves
(ACHR, 2004).

The current intra-Indigenous violence is perhaps alleviating pressure on the
Indigenous-settler conflict over political rights and natural resources, and is
weakening the Indigenous people in a number of ways. Since the intra-Indigenous
conflict is largely concentrated in Chakma inhabited areas, it is mostly the
Chakma who are the direct victims of violence, but other ethnic groups are also
affected due to restrictions on travel, pressure on business people and ordinary
people to pay 'contributions,' and so forth. Indigenous CHT society is therefore becoming increasingly divided, its economy is dwindling and its social and
human development through health care, education and training are stagnating
(Roy, 2000, 2003). Another factor was the lack of willingness of different successive governments to solve the problems of CHT conflict. Although successive
governments took several initiatives to resolve the problems, their intention was
not so clear. Before the Peace Accord was signed in 1997, no government treated
the CHT issue as a national issue; rather, the issue was tactfully kept away from
the national political agenda instead of anchored to national politics. On the other
hand, most of the government tried to solve the CHT conflict forcefully through
military, which created strong discontent among the Indigenous people in the
CHT. Increasing numbers of army forces were becoming a fashion for the government, which allowed the army to take control of the decision-making of this
region. Apart from above two factors, CHT conflict was banned from print and
news media before 1997 as issues of national security and concern. Thus, issues
relating to brutal torture of the Indigenous people by the army or the Bengali set-
ters did not draw the wider attention of the national or international community
before the peace treaty was signed.

Implementation of Peace Accord of 1997: The CHT Accord of 1997 promised
(i) land rights to the Indigenous people; (ii) revival of their cultural identities;
(iii) rehabilitation of internally displaced people and refugees who left the country;

(iv) withdrawal of military from the CHT, with the exception of permanent military establishments; (v) self-government through regional and district councils. These measures were a welcome relief from the more than 20 years of hostility and attacks on the Jumma people. Although most of the Indigenous communities viewed the accord as a step towards autonomy, voices within the PCJSS heavily criticized many aspects of it. Particularly scathing was the view expressed by a faction of its student organization—the faction later formed the UPDF—which described the accord as a 'sell-out.' Notwithstanding, the peace accord enhanced the image of the Bangladesh government in the international arena and earned then Prime Minister Sheikh Hasina the UNESCO Peace Prize in 1999. The accord speaks to four major issues in the CHT: (i) the devolution of power to the Hill District Councils, Regional Councils and the CHT Ministry as the units of self-government in the CHT; (ii) the establishment of a land commission to deal with conflicts over land and natural resource rights; (iii) recognition of the cultural integrity of the Indigenous peoples and the CHT as a 'tribal' area; and, finally, (iv) the withdrawal of military forces from CHT and the de-commissioning and rehabilitation of JSS forces. Although the government has amended existing laws to provide for the implementation of the peace accord, the accord faces a number of difficulties that require urgent and continued attention.

Although a decade has passed since the signing of the CHT Peace Accord on 2 December 1997, discontent persists in the region because the government has not fully implemented it. The accord ended two decades of bush war and sought to make the Indigenous people happy by involving them in the local administration, but their participation in the decision-making process still remains negligible. The hill people are unhappy that the army presence in the region continues despite the peace accord; moreover, it has virtually divided the Indigenous people into two groups—one opposing it and the other still hoping it will be implemented in full. Since the accord was signed, over 500 people belonging to the two groups have been killed and more than 1,000 injured in clashes between them. About 1,000 people from the two groups have been kidnapped. The CHT region also witnesses a rise in extortion by local gangs backed by the feuding groups. Complaints about the government's non-implementation are numerous. J.B. Larma, president of the JSS and current chairperson of the CHT Regional Council, has repeatedly complained, and in no uncertain terms, about non-implementation of the accord.

The Hill District Councils (HDC): The accord strengthens the power and authority of the 1989 HDCs. They are to be responsible for as many as 33 issues, including primary education and health, land and natural resources, development, environment and fisheries. Composed of 34 members with a 2/3 Indigenous majority (1/3 are to be from among the Bengalis), the HDCs are currently functional with five members each.

Establishment of a Regional Council (RC): The 22-member Regional Council is an apex body and plays a supervisory and coordinative role over HDCs, civil administration and the CHT Development Board. In 1991, an interim RC was established with the chairperson and majority of its members appointed from amongst the PCJSS nominees. The CHT Regional Council Act of 1998 is yet to be substantially implemented to enable the RC to play its supervisory and coordinative role while its legislative prerogatives are yet to be tested.

Recognition of Customary Rights: The land commission is to adjudicate land claims taking into account customary land laws. A highly controversial Land Disputes Resolution Act was passed by the previous government in July 2001, giving final deciding powers to the Chairman of the Land Commission regarding land disputes. The Regional Council has criticized the 2001 Act as giving wide-ranging and arbitrary powers to the commissioner and has proposed 18 amendments to the Act (Dictaan-Bang-oa Eleanor, 2004).

Land Administration Authority: Only primary education, social welfare and health were transferred to the HDCs. Land, land management and security/police, which are crucial in the CHT problem, have not been devolved to the local level. An office has been established in Khagrachari district, but the other members of the commission including the HDC and RC, the traditional rajas/kings have not been formally appointed. As of May 2003, some 35,000 cases had been filed, involving land disputes between the Indigenous peoples and the state-sponsored settlers (Dictaan-Bang-oa Eleanor, 2004). Although the Accord recognizes the CHT as a "tribal-inhabited area," this has not been recognized by legislation. So far, the HDCs and the RCs have not framed any subsidiary laws for the Indigenous peoples of the CHT. Indigenous languages in Bangladesh are facing threat due to government negligence and existing government frameworks were limited to starting multilingual education. Bangladesh is yet to recognize languages of the Indigenous communities in the country. Several government frameworks to protect them are moving slowly. In Bangladesh, there are about 40 languages. According to a report by Save the Children UK, Bangladesh Programme, a joint publication of Khagrachhari Hill District Council, Zabarang Kalyan Samity, and Save the Children, identified Tripura, Chakma, Marma, Achik (garo), Sadri (Oraon), Santal language as endangered language (Hasan, 2016).

Europe: Since much is not known about Indigenous peoples in contemporary Europe, I will focus on the Saami in brief. The Saami,[5] Indigenous peoples in Finland, have had the right to use the Saami language before public authorities since 1992. This right has been enshrined in the Constitution since 1995. At the beginning of 2004, the linguistic rights of the Saami were strengthened by the entry into force by a new Saami Language Act (Tebtebba, 2004). This Act applies to all courts and other public authorities operating within the Saami homeland, in the municipalities of Enontekiö, Inari and Utsjoki in the northern part of Finland, and in the reindeer owners' association of Lapland situated within the municipality of Sodankylä. The Act guarantees the use of all the Saami languages spoken in Finland: Inari Saami, Skolt Saami and Northern Saami. The Act lays down a duty for the authorities to, on their own initiative, see to it that the linguistic rights of the Saami are enforced. The Government report on the application of the language legislation, which is given to the Parliament for each of its terms on the basis of the Language Act, must also clarify the implementation of the provisions concerning the use of the Saami language before the authorities (Dictaan-Bang-oa, 2004).

Notes

1. Alberta is the only province that has passed legislation specifically for Métis people. On November 1, 1990 the Government of Alberta proclaimed legislation that provides for a unique form of government on the Métis Settlements. Developed cooperatively by the Province of Alberta and the Alberta Federation of Métis Settlements Association, this legislation establishes the only Métis land base and the only form of legislated Métis government in Canada. It was created in an effort to accommodate Métis aspirations of securing their land base, gaining local autonomy and achieving self-sufficiency (Aboriginal Affairs and Northern Development, 2008). The legislation consists of: Métis Settlements Act; Métis Settlements Land Protection Act; Constitution of Alberta Amendment Act, 1990; Métis Settlements Accord Implementation Act. These Acts establish the constitutional protection of 1.25 million acres of Settlement lands, the development of local government structures and systems, and provincial financial commitments (Aboriginal Affairs and Northern Development, 2008).
2. The issue of Nunavut, a project to create a self-governing territory in the eastern and northern portions of the Northwest Territories, is significant in the debate of self-government in Canada (Jull, 1988). Though the most ambitious of the Canadian aboriginal proposals for self-government, it combines Canadian traditions of social and political philosophy with the needs of Inuit culture.
3. In the Mixed Member Proportional (MMP) system, in existence since 1993, there are seven Maori seats, elected only by Maori electors on the Maori roll.
4. Some Maori political movements have advocated for *tino rangatiratanga*—that is, a degree of self-determination consistent with the Treaty of Waitangi. In consultation with Maori, both central Government and the Law Commission are considering options for improving the forms of legal entities available to Maori for governance purposes.
5. Approximately 11,000 people have registered in the Saami electoral roll, which comprises a list of all Saami people over the age of 18 who have registered to vote and take part in elections to the Sámediggi (Saami Parliament).

6 Policies, Governance and International Processes

UN Permanent Forum on Indigenous Issues

After about two decades of relentless efforts of the Indigenous peoples in the United Nations system, the UNHRC adopted the UN Declaration on the Rights of Indigenous Peoples (UDRIP). The United Nations Permanent Forum on Indigenous Issues (Permanent Forum) provides expert advice to the United Nations Economic and Social Council (ECOSOC) and to other agencies of the United Nations programs. The Permanent Forum has become one of three United Nations bodies that are mandated to deal specifically with causes of Indigenous peoples. The Permanent Forum holds a two-week session at the UN Headquarters during April or May, which offers windows for Indigenous peoples to engage in direct dialogue with members of the Forum and Human Rights Special Rapporteurs, other expert bodies and Member States (The Indigenous World, 2013).

In order to develop a set of minimum standards to protect Indigenous peoples the UN Economic and Social Council (ECOSOC) established the Working Group on Indigenous Populations (WGIP) in 1982. In fact, the increasingly reported oppression, marginalization and exploitation suffered by Indigenous peoples resulted in establishment of such group. WGIP submitted a first draft declaration on the rights of Indigenous peoples to the Sub-Commission on the Prevention of Discrimination and Protection of Minorities, which was later approved in 1994 (Martínez-Cobo, 1987).

The Permanent Forum holds an annual international expert group meetings. Participants are from the seven socio-cultural regions who present on topics relevant to global interest. The most recent past meeting was held at the UN Headquarters in 2012 on combating violence against Indigenous women and girls. Indigenous women and girls are exposed to diverse forms of physical, psychological and sexual violence. Indigenous women and girls face varied forms of discriminations specific to Indigenous identity and culture that are barriers to the capacity and potential of Indigenous peoples to exercise their rights. One of the most important tasks of the experts was to point out these various forms of discriminations, which have long-term implications to access to civic opportunities such as education, health care and justice (The Indigenous World, 2013).

The UNDRIP has been particular about the state's obligation to protect Indigenous women and girls from violence. However, states often are reluctant to pay heed to the need for better understanding and addressing violence against Indigenous women and girls. "Participants at the expert group meeting called upon the United Nations system, Member States and Indigenous peoples' organizations to recognize the rights and special needs of Indigenous women and girls" (The Indigenous World, 2013: 450).

It is worth mentioning the 11th Session of the Permanent Forum on Indigenous Issues primarily because of its significance in terms of the role played in recognizing the rights of the Indigenous population. This session took a different and very important shape due to the presence of more than 1,200 Indigenous peoples' representatives, some 50 Member States, UN system agencies, funds and programs, and NGOs. The Doctrine of Discovery was one of the themes discussed in the 11th session "in light of the legal and political justification for the dispossession of Indigenous peoples from their lands, their disenfranchisement and the abrogation of their rights, Indigenous peoples were constructed as 'savages,' 'barbarians,' 'backward' and 'inferior and uncivilized' by the colonizers, who used such constructs to subjugate, dominate and exploit Indigenous peoples" (The Indigenous World, 2013: 451). As it has interest in the work, the Permanent Forum had an in-depth dialogue with the World Intellectual Property Organization (WIPO), focusing many areas of Indigenous peoples. In order to mark the fifth anniversary of the adoption of the UNDRIP, the UN General Assembly held a high-level commemorative event at the UN Headquarters, which was addressed by the UN Secretary-General, the President of the UN General Assembly, the Minister for Foreign Affairs of the Plurinational State of Bolivia, representatives of Indigenous Peoples' caucuses and several governments that emphasized that the UNDRIP had become a unique international instrument on a range of issues and set standards that would be the foundation for the continued survival of Indigenous peoples and protection of their dignity and wellbeing (The Indigenous World, 2013).

UN World Conference

The conference was held from 22 to 23 September 2014. The Third Committee of the United Nations General Assembly adopted a resolution to organize a high-level plenary meeting of the General Assembly (GA), the World Conference on Indigenous Peoples. The primary aim of the conference was to pursue the objectives of the United Nations Declaration on the Rights of Indigenous Peoples (UNPFII, 2014).

This was the first UN meeting ever at this level that focused solely on Indigenous peoples' rights. This has generated huge expectations among global policy makers in general and Indigenous peoples in particular. There has been though doubts and skepticism about the outcome of the meeting. Many initiatives have been developed by the Indigenous peoples to ensure the participation in relevant meetings, including both the preparatory and post Conference processes. This was possible primarily due to the GA resolution (The Indigenous World, 2013). In early 2012, a brainstorming meeting with Indigenous peoples was held in

Copenhagen on the conference. The Copenhagen meeting ended up with a resolution that recognizing that maintaining the UN Declaration on the Rights of Indigenous Peoples as standard was important. Again, in mid 2013 another meeting was held in Norway for the Indigenous peoples to be able to consolidate their strategies and inputs. They wrote a concept paper that outlined significant points they felt need attention.

As I mentioned elsewhere in the book about the Indigenous Global Coordinating Group (GCG), lobbies for the full and effective participation of Indigenous peoples in the preparatory processes led up to and continued during and after the meeting (The Indigenous World, 2013). In 2012, the GA set out a framework (i.e. the date, number of plenary sessions, opening and closing sessions, roundtable and informal sessions for the conference). That GA as well set out the potential participants. The resolution made sure that Indigenous participation at all level of the conference was ensured. Indigenous peoples found this conference as an opportunity for them to raise awareness of their rights and push for their greater recognition. However, a lot of skepticisms were there about the end result.

UN Special Rapporteur on Indigenous Peoples

It is widely believed that Indigenous peoples face discrimination because of their distinct cultures, identities and ways of life all over the world. This is as well the consequences of historical colonization and invasion of their territories (UNPFII, 2014). The international community has begun to pay attention to the human rights situations of Indigenous peoples.

The Special Rapporteur on the Rights of Indigenous Peoples has the mandate to gather information and communications from all relevant sources on violations of human rights of Indigenous peoples, based on which, the Special Rapporteur can receive and investigate complaints from Indigenous individuals, groups or communities; undertake country visits; and make recommendations to governments on steps needed to remedy possible violations or to prevent future violations (OHCHR, 2015). The Special Rapporteur offers technical support to state governments and agencies regarding Indigenous peoples through making comments to draft regulations on Indigenous consultation and participation developed by the various governments (The Indigenous World, 2013).

The Special Rapporteur examines specific cases of alleged human rights violations and, as a result, urgent appeal letters are issued to governments on human situations.

In 2012, the Special Rapporteur sent communications on situations in Argentina, Australia, Brazil, Cameroon, Chile, Colombia, Costa Rica, Guatemala, Ethiopia, Finland, Indonesia, Kenya, Mexico, Nepal, New Zealand, Panama, Peru, Philippines, Russian Federation, Suriname, United States and Venezuela. In various cases examined, the Special Rapporteur issued follow-up communications and observations. These included, for example, the situation of Indigenous peoples affected by the Phulbari coal mine in Bangladesh; the situation of Indigenous protests against a proposed road construction project through the TIPNIS reserve in Bolivia; the social and economic conditions of the Attawapiskat First Nation in Canada; the human rights effects of the Gibe III hydroelectric dam in Ethiopia; the situation of alleged diminishment of Saami self-determination resulting from a decision by the Finland Supreme Administrative Court; the social conflicts surrounding the construction of a cement plant in the predominantly Indigenous municipality of San Juan Sacatepéquez, Guatemala; and the health situation of Leonard Peltier, an Indigenous activist in the United States serving consecutive life sentences in prison.

(The Indigenous World, 2013: 460)

The Phulbari Coal Mine project affected around half million people and most of the immediately affected are Indigenous population.

The Special Rapporteur in 2012 visited a number of countries, such as Argentina, the USA, El Salvador and Namibia, and prepared assessment reports. The Special Rapporteur urged the government of El Salvador to establish participatory mechanisms for Indigenous peoples within the decision-making framework of the state. For the United States, the Special Rapporteur noted the need to address persistent, deep-seated problems arising from historical wrongs towards reconciliation with Indigenous peoples. In his press statement on concluding his Namibia visit, the Special Rapporteur noted the need for greater inclusion of Indigenous minority groups at all levels of decision-making, for full recognition of their traditional authorities, and for a strengthening of their rights to lands and natural resources. In Argentina, main issues covered in the report included land and natural resource rights, extractive and commercial agricultural activities, the eviction of Indigenous communities and the socioeconomic concerns of Indigenous peoples (The Indigenous World, 2013).

The Special Rapporteur called for the need for a holistic approach to protect the rights of Indigenous women and children by way of implementing the declaration on the rights of Indigenous peoples within programs targeting violence against Indigenous women and girls. The Special Rapporteur attaches emphasis to the substantive rights of Indigenous peoples, which include rights to lands and natural resources, culture, religion, health and the pursuit of their own development priorities and self-determination. "In this sense, efforts to prevent and punish violence against Indigenous women and girls must also work towards enhancing Indigenous self-determination and cultural integrity" (The Indigenous World, 2013: 462).

UN Human Rights Council

The United Nations Human Rights Council (HRC), created in 2006 by the UN GA, promotes and provides protection of human rights around the world. The HRC is constituted by 47 United Nations Member States, which are elected by the UN General Assembly. The Human Rights Council works with the UN special rapporteurs established by the former Commission on Human Rights and now assumed by the Council. These are made up of special rapporteurs, special representatives, independent experts and working groups that monitor, examine, advise and publicly report on thematic issues or human rights situations in specific countries. The Human Rights Council meets three times a year for three weeks in Geneva (OHCHR, 2014; United Nations, 2014).

The Human Rights Council (HRC) in the 21st ordinary session turned its attention to the rights of Indigenous peoples. There was a panel in the session that considered the issue of Indigenous peoples and access to justice. In this session, the Special Rapporteur (SR) gave a briefing on the visits to the USA, Argentina and El Salvador, along with two major issues: violence against Indigenous women and girls and the impact of the extractive industries on Indigenous rights. The SR's report clearly shows that problem of violence against women and children could not be dissociated from the marginalization and oppression Indigenous peoples suffer. The Chair of the EMRIP presented findings of a study on the role of languages and culture in promoting and protecting the rights and identity of Indigenous peoples, including the obstacles Indigenous peoples face to enjoying their right to their own culture (The Indigenous World, 2013: 466). Then the USA spoke recognizing the marginalization and disadvantage suffered by Native Americans in the USA. They, as well, explained that they are taking steps to remedy this situation by allocating larger budgets. Argentina also reported that there is impressive progress in the legislation in the country with regard to recognizing Indigenous rights.

Guatemala placed emphasis on the fact that there is a need to adopt a decision with regard to the Secretary-General's report on Indigenous peoples' participation at the United Nations of Indigenous peoples representatives.

> Mexico referred to the issues under consideration and affirmed the right of Indigenous peoples to self-determination and to preserve the integrity of their lands. The European Union underscored the importance of the issue of violence against Indigenous women; with regard to the extractive industries, it stated that it was placing particular emphasis on corporate social responsibility and that a new European policy had been adopted in this regard. In the second part of the interactive dialogue, Peru, Australia, Norway, Russia, Venezuela, Chile, Bolivia, Sweden and others all referred to the extractive industries, noting national progress and highlighting the importance of the framework of principles adopted by the Council in this regard. A number focused on the problem of violence against Indigenous women (Peru, Australia, Venezuela, Bolivia, Nepal, Finland, Paraguay, Austria, Malaysia). Brazil and Colombia noted the progress made on the issue of consultation and of their success in dialoguing with Indigenous peoples.
>
> (The Indigenous World, 2013: 467)

It is worth a mention that since 2012 an expert panel on issues related to the rights of Indigenous peoples has been organized in the official HRC session. In the first expert panel in 2012, all the speakers emphasized Indigenous peoples' difficulties with regard to accessing national justice systems and getting their own systems of law and justice to be recognized.

Business and Human Rights: The Human Rights Council endorsed the Guiding Principles on Business and Human Rights: Implementing the United Nations "Protect, Respect and Remedy—the first ever precedence that a UN intergovernmental body endorsed a normative document on the previously divisive issue of business and human rights" (The Indigenous World, 2013: 471). The Council appointed five experts for three years as members of a Working Group, which was formed in January 2012. The Group meets three times a year in closed sessions, and it has responsibility for organizing a yearly Forum on Business and Human Rights.

The Working Group organized stakeholder meetings at the UN in Geneva, which provided general information about its mandate and its work plan. The importance of focusing on Indigenous peoples and local communities was one of the themes of the meetings. In 2012, another Working Group meeting with Indigenous experts and members of the UN permanent forum was organized in which challenges regarding the implementation of the UN Guiding Principles with regards to Indigenous peoples and possible further plans were discussed.

The Working Group is going to declare the issue of Indigenous peoples a priority in the work of the implementation of the Guiding Principles and to prepare its first thematic report to the UN General Assembly in 2013 on the topic of Indigenous peoples' human rights and business. The Working Group in the first annual Forum on Business and Human Rights organized a panel discussion where "participants expressed their concerns with the perceived weakness of existing remedies and emphasized that Indigenous peoples are collective rights-holders under international law, entitled to self-determination and pointed out the pivotal importance of the concept of Free, Prior and Informed Consent (FPIC), stemming from this right" (The Indigenous World, 2013: 472).

Peace Agreements in Chittagong Hill Tract: Indigenous people are called in various terms in Bangladesh. However, one of the most used terms is 'Upojati,' which literally means 'sub-nation,' and another is 'Adibashi,' which means 'Indigenous' or 'Aboriginals'(Dhamai, 2006; Roy, 2010). Most of them are concentrated on Chittagong Hill area, while some others are scattered in plain lands.

These people, like those elsewhere in the world, have been struggling to obtain autonomy and to protect themselves from human rights violations. Longstanding problems have existed related to the fact that their way of life has been encroached by government policy of allowing non-Indigenous people to grab their lands. Their region was militarized. This often led them to engage in violent insurgencies. With a view to ending such problems in 1997, a "Peace Accord" was signed between the National Committee on Chittagong Hill Tracts and the *Parbhatia Chttagram Jana Sanghati Samiti* (PCJSS) in the presence of highest government authorities in Bangladesh (Hossain, 2013). However, due to the lack of political commitment, implementation of the Peace Accord remained uncertain. Claims exist that the Peace Accord was not signed with the consent of other major political parties because the government wanted to take all the credit for this endeavor. The national Committee on CHT Affairs, on behalf of the Bangladesh government and the PCJSS, on behalf of the inhabitants of the Chittagong Hill Tracts, arrived at an agreement in order to elevate sociopolitical, cultural, educational and financial rights of all citizens in CHT.

World Heritage Convention: In 1972 the General Conference of the UNESCO adopted a multilateral treaty—one of the most accepted international instruments—on the protection of the world cultural and natural heritage. The primary idea of the Convention is that some natural and cultural heritage is so important that its protection is not only the responsibility of the states but also a duty of the international community. The World Heritage Committee (WHC), consisting of 21 States Parties, maintains a World Heritage List and ensures that the sites are adequately protected for future generations.

Rio + 20: In June 2012, the Rio + 20 conference that took place in Rio de Janeiro was attended by a huge number of Indigenous representatives. They engaged in official negotiations with governments, business, NGOs. They also organized a few event events such as the Kari-Oca II, the World Indigenous Peoples' Conference on Territories, Rights and Sustainable Development (The Indigenous World, 2013). Over 500 Indigenous leaders signed the Kari-Oca II Declaration, which was subsequently delivered to the Brazilian government.

"The Campamento Tierra Libre y Vida Plena held during the Peoples' Summit brought together Indigenous representatives from the Amazon region to call for recognition of Indigenous peoples' rights to land, territories and resources and to reject the increasing encroachment onto their land by the extractive industries, in collaboration with national governments" (The Indigenous World, 2013: 487). The Indigenous Peoples' International Conference, organized by the Global Coordination Committee, on Sustainable Development met with the goal of sharing Indigenous peoples' experiences, perspectives and practices with regard to sustainable development.

UN Framework Convention on Climate Change (UNFCCC)

The rights of Indigenous peoples intersect almost all areas of negotiation but have been demonstrated prominently within the negotiations on forest conservation, known as REDD+ (Reduced Emissions from Deforestation and Forest Degradation). The bigger picture and main developments are in the UNFCCC. The 18th COP, which took place in December 2012 in Doha, Qatar, laid out the roadmap for the negotiations towards a globally binding agreement on emissions reductions.

The third main issue of negotiation in Doha was the operationalization of the ADP, which was negotiated at COP17 in Durban in 2011 and represents the key negotiation path for a new binding agreement on emission reductions in 2015—effective from 2020. Indigenous peoples need to highlight and underscore this innovative and extraordinary reference to international instruments, such as the UNDRIP, in any outcome document of the ADP.

In fact, Indigenous people have already stressed three pillars on which any climate programme and policy should be based, notably: 1. Recognition of the rights of Indigenous peoples in accordance with international standards and instruments such as the UNDRIP, including Free, Prior and Informed Consent; 2. Respect for traditional knowledge and recognition of the key role of Indigenous people in adaptation and mitigation; 3. Respect for Indigenous peoples' right to full and effective participation. Indigenous peoples have always stressed that all aspects of climate change and climate change measures—adaptation, mitigation—are ultimately rights issues, as they directly affect their lives and livelihoods. A human rights-based approach is therefore crucial and their demands are key to their involvement. It is therefore positive to note that a number of actors in the UNFCCC context have started to raise human rights issues.

(The Indigenous World, 2014: 493)

For Canada, with few prospects for constitutional change following the 1992 referendum, the Liberal government elected in 1993 committed itself to recognizing the inherent right of self-government and implement it without reopening constitutional discussions. In August 1995, the federal government formally announced its new policy. Key principles of the policy are (Wherrett, 1999):

- the inherent right is an existing Indigenous right under section 35 of the *Constitution Act, 1982*.
- self-government will be exercised within the existing Canadian constitution.
- the *Canadian Charter of Rights and Freedoms* will apply to Indigenous governments.
- federal funding for self-government will be achieved through the reallocation of existing resources.
- where all parties agree, rights in self-government agreements may be protected in new treaties under section 35 of the Constitution, as additions to existing treaties, or as part of comprehensive land claims agreements.
- laws of overriding federal and provincial importance will prevail, and federal, provincial, territorial and Indigenous laws must work in harmony.

Under this policy, the range of subjects that the federal government is willing to negotiate includes matters internal to the group, integral to Indigenous culture, and essential to operating as a government or institution. Examples are the establishment of government structures and internal constitutions; membership; marriage; Indigenous languages, culture and religion; education; health; social services; policing; enforcement of Indigenous laws; and others.

Stages in Norwegian Saami Policy: Norwegian government policy towards the Saami has changed through the centuries, both in accordance with international trends, and in terms of national interests. In order to provide a context, we sketch some major trends in Norwegian government policy towards the Saami minority since 1850. At that point, there was a change in the policy with the introduction of the so-called Norwegianization policy, which was active until 1959. We demonstrate three stages of governmental policy: Norwegianization/ assimilation, 1850–1959; economic and cultural integration, or integrated pluralism, 1959–1984; and cultural pluralism, 1984 to the present.

The European Union plays a major role in international cooperation and norms and policy setting in establishing policies on the rights of Indigenous peoples. Looking at the internal aspects, the principles of liberty, democracy, respect for human rights and fundamental freedoms and the rule of law are inherent to the European integration process. The calls for these policies have their roots in external and internal demands and norms vis-à-vis human rights under which the now widely recognized norms for the rights of Indigenous peoples have developed. The EU fosters the universality and indivisibility of all human rights—civil, political, economic, social and cultural—as stipulated in the Universal Declaration of Human Rights and reaffirmed by the World Conference on Human Rights.

Select Evidence of Self-Governance

Governments of most countries with Indigenous peoples tend to find ways for them to have more involvement in decision-making that affect their health and economy. Academics, political leaders, and government representatives express their opinion and concern about the most beneficial structure of self-government, about who controls what, about when self-government should be implemented, about whether or not a true form of self-government can ever be achieved. Hereunder some cases of self-government have been provided to demonstrate how this self-government has affected health of the Indigenous peoples.

Self-governance and the case of Bolivia: While most Indigenous peoples favor a move to self-governance, the current level of self-governance varies from country to country. Greenland, with its Home Rule Government, the formation of the new territory of Nunavut in Canada and the Norwegian Saami Parliament are the most advanced examples (AMAP, 1997). In the Russian Federation, the Russian Association of Indigenous Peoples of the North, Far East and Siberia is working to link 30 Indigenous minority groups and present a united voice to official, Moscow-led, governance (Scarpa, 2013). NGOs are connecting Indigenous peoples across national boundaries. The Arctic Council, the intergovernmental process towards sustainable development in the Arctic, has established an Indigenous Peoples Secretariat to support and coordinate the activities of the Indigenous participants to the process (AMAP, 1997).

Indigenous peoples continually find themselves subordinated within the nation-state and international system and, as a consequence, their standards of living have had to be raised through the cracks left open, by unexpected events and the passage of time, in the oppressors' own discourses and legal expressions of rights. Evo Morales, an Aymara Indian with a bootstrap story of childhood poverty and the backing of much of the nation's poor and Indigenous population, scored a solid win in his race for president. Evo Morales, a successor of Eduardo Rodriguez (9 June 2005 – 22 January 2006) has been in power since 22 January

2006) was part of a wave of leftists taking power in Latin America and rejecting Washington's neoliberal economic policies. Carlos Mesa (whose predecessor was Eduardo Rodriguez) came to power in October 2003 after a wave of demonstrations left almost 100 dead and forced his predecessor to flee the country. Less than two years later, in March 2005, he was driven from office by his inability to meet the demands of either the Indigenous movements, the business sector, or wealthy provinces looking for more autonomy. Since then Supreme Court president Eduardo Rodriguez had held a tenuous grip on the highest office, succeeding Carlos Mesa, who had resigned among mass protests and road blockades that paralyzed the country for weeks (Foek, 2005).

Morales's election affects the crucial battle to control Bolivia's resources. In the past, as former president Mesa noted, the winners in Bolivia have been transnational corporations from Brazil, Argentina, the United States, China and Mexico and Europe. Petrobras of Brazil, Repsol YPF of Spain, the French Total, British Gas and British Petroleum and scores of others, among them the Royal Dutch Shell, have been granted broad access to Bolivia's resources to take most of the profits home, which have been vast. The country is still rich in tin reserves, silver, zinc, timber, water, oil, and natural gas. Many of the Indigenous people do not have the legal right to live on the lands they depend on for survival or to use the resources they have managed on a sustainable basis for thousands of years (Craib et al., 2003). Outsiders (i.e. non-Indigenous) increasingly exploit resources, with few benefits flowing to Indigenous communities and with little regard for the natural environment. However, Indigenous people are often held responsible for exploitation of the natural resources that poor countries must undertake in order to participate in the global economy and raise their standard of living. The process is occurring with lethal effects in Bangladesh, India, Indonesia, Brazil and other parts of the world. Indigenous resources have given rise to the development of new drugs. The significant examples of how Indigenous Australian knowledge of plants has been used in this way include Duboisia, a plant from Queensland and northern New South Wales, found to contain hyoscine, which has been used as a sedative in treating motion sickness and as a truth serum (Janke, n.d.).

In Bangladesh, for example, women who are Indigenous experience discrimination and racism from the dominant culture and nation-state. On one hand, their status as Indigenous people is not recognized by the state within which they find themselves. Their mobility is very much confined within their own community. Therefore, their livelihood is based on natural resources, and they don't have access to employment. Thus the natural scape in Chittagong is at stake because of overexploitation (Cholchester, 1995: 59).

Diverse development projects undertaken in the Indigenous community were based on the use of natural resources. For example, a factory to process palm-sprouts was opened in an area where a businessman showed up wanting to cut down every single palm in the forest for the palm hearts. Businesspeople did that without any resistance from the Indigenous community, and that was how the destruction of the palm forest began (Blaser et al., 2008). Palms have been very important to the Indigenous as they use them as food, as medicine for hepatitis and parasites, and as material for their houses. The leaders got together and calculated that the 600 guaranis (US$0.25) that would be paid for each sprout did not begin to cover the total value of the palm trees in terms of food, medicine, construction materials and handicrafts. Without palm trees they have no reserve of food, no medicine, no houses. Ultimately, they were able to save the palm trees (Barras, 2004).

Self-governance of Saami in Norway: The Saami people, the most significant ethnic minority in Scandinavia, in the 1980s were granted a constitutional right to preserve their culture in Norway. Earlier this year the Norwegian parliament passed a law that went further than that, granting the Saami people special property rights in the northernmost province of Finnmark, over that of Norwegian citizens of non-Saami origin.

The Saami Parliament is an Indigenous electoral body elected among and for the Saami people in Norway. The Saami Parliament, representing the Saami people in all matters concerning them, has its separate electoral system with elections every fourth year. Norway has constitutionally recognized the Saami as an Indigenous people. The Saamis' right to self-determination according to Article 1 of the UN Covenants on Civil and Political Rights and Economical, Social and Cultural Rights are, however, not yet fully acknowledged by Norway (Sara, 2006). Two progressive steps towards Indigenous Governance in Norway, namely the recent adoption of the Finnmark Act and the legislative adoption of the recent Agreement on Consultation Procedures between the Government and the Executive Council of the Saami Parliament, are worth mentioning. The Saami people are one people in four different countries, Norway, Sweden, Finland and Russia, of which each of the first three countries has Saami Parliaments. This is how the Saami of Norway, Sweden and Finland have chosen to resolve the lack of or under representation of Saami in the national and regional electoral bodies (Sara, 2006).

The Saamis' right to develop the Saami languages and culture was officially recognized in the 1960s, and later, in 1989, the Saamis' political rights were recognized by the establishment of the Saami Parliament. In 1988 the Norwegian Parliament passed a new act inspired by the UN covenant on Civil and Political rights. The Constitutional Act 110a provides recognition and protection of the Saamis language, culture and society. Norway also ratified the ILO Convention no. 169 as the first country in 1990. Even though the ILO Convention was ratified, it would take 15 years before the first broad effort of implementation would take place through the adoption of the Finnmark Act. This was also the first time substantial consultations according to article 6 of the ILO Convention 169 were carried out between the Norwegian Parliament and the Saami Parliament (Tebtebba, 2004).

Métis Settlements and Nunavut in Canada: Federal and provincial governments want Indigenous peoples to be involved in health policymaking processes (Wall, 1998). Critics of current forms of Aboriginal self-government view them as little more than convenient arrangements that allow Aboriginal people administrative responsibility for services which are ultimately controlled by the federal or provincial government (Dacks, 1986). Self-government proposals also have their critics among the very people for whom they are intended. For example, Inuit women have objected to many parts of the Nunavut agreement mainly because of concerns about an emphasis on conventional southern Canadian notions of resource management. They also had concerns about an emphasis on the economic, social and political roles and issues for men at the expense of those of women in Nunavut (Inuit Women's Association, 1993). Although there are differences between these two contemporary forms of self-government (the Alberta Métis Settlements Accords and agreements of the late 1980s and to Nunavut), there are similarities (Inuit Women's Association, 1993).

One major difference between these two forms of Aboriginal self-government is that the Alberta Métis Settlements Councils are clear examples of ethnic governments that are elected and operated by members of a particular ethnic group. The Métis Settlements Accord led to Royal Assent of four pieces of Alberta legislation in November 1990. These established land ownership rights and a reorganized form of governance for the Métis of the eight Alberta Settlements. With the introduction of land claims policies of the Federal government and the Trudeau government acceptance of the notions of Aboriginal rights, following the Nisga'a Case of 1973, Canadian comprehensive land claims began in earnest (Wall, 1998). Since then, specific and comprehensive claims have piled up on the federal doorstep by many. One of these claims was the 1976 Inuit claim over eastern Arctic lands. That claims settlement resulted in Nunavut, Canada's third Territory stretching from Hudson Bay to the northernmost parts of Ellesmere Island. Under the terms of the settlement, the government of Nunavut has powers like those of other Territorial governments, established and maintained in the context of a very close working relationship with the Federal government (Inuit Women's Association, 1993; Wall, 1998).

The Finnmark Act: The basic tenet of the Finnmark Act is that the management of land and natural resources in Finnmark County shall focus especially on securing Saami culture, reindeer husbandry, rough pasturing, economic activity and community life. This basic premise and the recognition of Saami rights in principle constitute the very essence of the Finnmark Act and will have an effect on comparable processes involving the rights of the Saami and other Indigenous peoples in other areas and other countries. The Finnmark Act establishes a new autonomous organization for the administration of land, water and resources in Finnmark called the Finnmark Estate. According to the act, the Saami Parliament appoints half of the board members, and these board members in principle have the deciding vote in matters concerning changed use of the uncultivated areas of the innermost part of Finnmark. The Saami Parliament is also to provide guidelines regarding considerations that are to be taken by state, county and municipal authorities when making changes in the use of uncultivated areas. As regards whether or not to permit the mining of claimable minerals in Finnmark County, great importance should be attached to consideration for Saami culture, including industries and rough pasturing. The scope of the act is also limited to Finnmark County, which is only a part of the traditional Saami territories in Norway (Sara, 2006).

The agreement on consultation procedures: In addition to the Finnmark Act, there is another step, which is the agreement on consultation procedures. The Saami Parliament emphasizes that the Storting has taken Norway's obligation under international law about consulting with the Saami people in connection with the drafting of the Finnmark Act seriously, and that this is new, relative to the country's constitution. The Saami Parliament would also call attention to the fact that the consultations have been very useful in the efforts to arrive at a proposal that was acceptable to the Saami Parliament.

The Norwegian State also adopted the Agreement into national legislation in 2005.[1] The agreement is intended to acknowledge the Norwegian State's obligations under international law to consult with the Indigenous peoples on any legislation and measures that can have a direct impact on the Saami. Consultations shall be conducted before decisions are adopted. In particular, Article 6 of ILO Convention No. 169 regarding Indigenous and Tribal Peoples in Independent Countries calls for such consultations. Other provisions in ILO Convention No. 169 as well as Articles 1 and 27 of the UN Covenant on Civil and Political Rights are also of significance in this context.

Consultations were carried out on several occasions after this, and while there are still many unsolved questions and differences between the parties regarding the extent of the agreement, the relationship between the Saami Parliament and the government has been moving towards a mutual partnership in the consultations procedures. The ultimate decisions are, however still made by the state (Sara, 2006). As a result, a wave of constitutional reforms incorporating Indigenous claims started with Nicaragua in 1987, continued with Brazil (1988), Colombia (1991), Paraguay (1992), Mexico (1992), Peru (1993), Argentina (1994), Bolivia (1994), and Panama (1994) (Sara, 2006). The last two and most comprehensive amendments have been the Ecuadorian (1998) and Venezuelan (1999) reforms (UN, 2006).

Policies in Asia: The CHT Peace Accord signed between the government and Indigenous Jumma peoples in 1997 introduces a special political arrangement for CHT with the formation of CHT Regional Council (CHTRC) as an apex political body of the region and the three Hill District Councils (HDCs). The newly introduced CHT Regional Council and the somewhat older Hill District Councils are also unique to the CHT. The majority of the seats (two-thirds) in the CHTRC and HDCs, including the positions of the chairs, are reserved for Indigenous peoples and one-third of the seats are for permanent Bengali residents. The Peace Accord also contributed to the creation of the Ministry of Chittagong Hill Tracts Affairs (MoCHTA) in Dhaka, with a minister to be appointed from among the Indigenous peoples and for an Advisory Committee to be constituted to lend support to the ministry.

However, the PCJSS always kept the door open for a negotiated dialogue for resolving the CHT problem through political and peaceful means. Hence the formal dialogue was started in 1985 with the government. Finally, during the period of the Sheikh Hasina government on 2 December 1997, the CHT Accord, popularly known as CHT Peace Accord, was signed between the government and the PCJSS.

The Accord ends more than two decades of armed struggle for self-determination and paves the way for the peace, development and representation of the Jumma people. It recognizes the CHT as a tribal-inhabited region, and allowed for the establishment of the CHT Regional Council, the three Hill District Councils, the CHT Affairs Ministry and the Land Commission. It also sought the demilitarization of the region and the rehabilitation of the victims, among other things (AIPP, 2007). The government reserves 5 percent of the jobs in the Bangladesh Civil Service (BCS) for Indigenous peoples.

Note

1. On 11 May 2005, Minister of Local Government and Regional Development (the Minister in charge of Saami affairs for the Norwegian government) and the former President of the Saami Parliament signed an agreement regarding procedures for consultations between State authorities and the Saami Parliament in Norway.

7 Discussions and Policy Recommendations

Globalization has had disproportionate impact on Indigenous peoples worldwide, especially in some countries in the South. Therefore, global efforts in poverty reduction have not witnessed equitable change in poverty measures. Socioeconomic status measures are current income level, recent income change, poverty flags, current earnings, multi-period averaged incomes and relative position in the income distribution (Gurran and Phipps, 2003). Several studies demonstrate that there are associations between income and morbidity. Since the mid-nineteenth century, globalization has posed challenges for global health governance.

The right of self-determination of peoples is a fundamental principle in international law. It is embodied in the Charter of the United Nations and the International Covenant on Civil and Political Rights and the International Covenant on Economic, Social and Cultural Rights. The right of self-determination has been recognized in other international and regional human rights instruments, such as Part VII of the Helsinki Final Act 1975 and Article 20 of the African Charter of Human and Peoples' Rights, as well as the Declaration on the Granting of Independence to Colonial Territories and Peoples. By virtue of that right, Indigenous people are supposed to freely determine and pursue their political, economic, social and cultural roles in the society.

This book explores the importance of traditional activities for Indigenous peoples' health based on determinants of health framework. The research shows the significance of income, education and employment for health that is similar to other analyses of citizens in general, where a determinants of health framework has been employed. The inclusion of a subset of variables measuring traditional activities resulted in an attenuated set of meaningful results. In those countries where comparisons have been made between poverty levels of Indigenous peoples versus other population groups, poverty indicators point to large gaps. For example, in four countries in Latin America, during a decade in which overall poverty decreased, Indigenous peoples suffered not only higher poverty rates but also a widening gap from non-Indigenous peoples.

Chapter 2 deals with who and where the Indigenous are. There are widespread misunderstandings surrounding the definitions of *Indigenous*. While studies and researches are abundant on the Indigenous populations, no clear indication or estimate is so far available about their locations. This chapter provides an account of the Indigenous peoples around the world and offers definitions of *Indigenous*. Broadly, *Indigenous* refers to people comprising a group or culture regarded as coming from a given place; by this definition, this means almost any person or group is Indigenous to some location or other. As a contemporary cultural description, however, *Indigenous* has a much narrower common meaning, describing people who are regulated largely by their own traditions and customs. The most commonly used approaches to defining Indigenousness are language spoken, self-perception and geographic concentration. In order to protect Indigenous languages, governments must introduce multilingual education systems and facilitate opportunities for ethnic and Indigenous people to practice their culture in their own language. One Indigenous leader from Khagrachhori, Bangladesh, mentioned that the government is doing nothing except initiating a multilingual education system. Textbooks in Indigenous languages are yet to reach students. Indigenous communities arrange cultural programs to promote and protect their languages. But even the International Mother Language Institute has failed to create any effective project. Chapter 2 of the book attempts to arrive at a workable definition of Indigenous people (IP)—and, by extension, of non-IP—and a workable definition of "health"; it then provides a description, divided into regions, of numbers of IP, regional/global locations, and variations, with considerable detail on Eritrea and Bangladesh. The following chapter (chapter 3) is an attempt at providing a definition of SDH; the rationale for doing so; categorization into distal, intermediate and proximate; the complex graph is reduced, in the text, to the following SDHs—education, livelihoods and/or employment income, poverty, [structural] economic inequality, long-term stress, social exclusion, and longevity. Chapter 4 deals with how the exercise of rights, as enunciated in the UNDRIP, especially with respect to self-determination, has the potential to overcome the negative metrics of SDHs given in the previous chapter.

Chapter 5 begins with an attempt to relate self-determination (self-governance) to health. This is superseded by a world survey of "colonialism to self-governance" in Latin America, Canada, Australia-New Zealand, Bangladesh and Finland. Much of this material really belongs to the very political themes of the previous chapter.

Chapter 6 comprises sections on political themes about governance. It begins with a short description of the UN system and its agencies related to IP rights. This is followed by a description of recent processes of self-governance for IPs in the Chittagong Hill Tract. Then a description of the relevance of UNESCO World Heritage policies with respect to IPs. Then, IP representation at Rio + 20. Then IP input and association with the UNFCCC. Then a series of overviews on self-determination in Canada, Norway and Bolivia. This is followed by a short series of cameos regarding self- determination in Bangladesh, Norway (again), Canada (again), then Norway again (Finnmark region). This last chapter (chapter 7) summarizes the content of the preceding chapters; the last few sections attempt to begin a discussion of the whole IP problematic.

Indigenous peoples are generally regarded as the descendants of the original inhabitants of areas that have become occupied by more powerful outsiders, and whose language, culture and/or religion remain distinct from the dominant group. They are regarded as the inheritors and practitioners of unique ways of relating to other people and to the environment, retaining social, cultural, economic and political characteristics that are distinct from those of the dominant societies. At the same time, they also frequently suffer both discrimination and pressure to assimilate into their surrounding societies. And while a concern common to most Indigenous people is that their cultural uniqueness is being lost, dominant understandings of Indigenousness often conflate authenticity with objectification. 'Authentic' Indigenousness thus becomes defined by objective and observable traits (i.e. clothing and behaviors) that conform to the dominant definitions of what it is to be a member of this or that Indigenous population. When these traits are not portrayed, as is the case with Indigenous peoples in Paraguay, the authenticity of their claim to being Indigenous is regarded as 'inauthentic.' The same has been said of those Indigenous people who pursue economic and political goals that do not conform to dominant ideas of their Indigenousness.

Chapter three analyzes the interplay between globalization and social determinants of health of the Indigenous. This chapter grapples with the facts of health inequalities experienced by diverse Indigenous peoples in the world. The analysis includes the social determinants of health across the life course and provides evidence that not only demonstrates important health disparities within Indigenous groups and compared to non-Indigenous people, but also links social determinants—at proximal, intermediate and distal levels—to health inequalities. The increasing interconnectedness between societies has had an effect on economic growth since the early nineteenth century. Globalization processes, characterized by the increasing circulation of peoples, ideas and commodities, prompt the emergence of organizational forms that are intended to control, adapt and tap into those circulations. Thus, many of the functions held by the nation-state are transferred upwards to supranational institutions and common markets through economic and political integration, downwards to regions and communities through political and administrative decentralization, and sideways to NGOs and the private sector through 'democratization' and privatization.

Globalization appeared itself in many different forms, affecting almost the people of the world. A lot of attention is accorded to the extreme positive and negative impacts, globalization has generated. Similar results could be seen amongst the Indigenous peoples also. Little is known about the influence of social determinants of health in the lives of Indigenous peoples. Yet, it is clear that the physical, emotional, mental and spiritual dimensions of health among Indigenous children, youth and adults are distinctly, as well as differentially, influenced by a broad range of social determinants. These include circumstances and environments as well as structures, systems and institutions that influence the development and maintenance of health along a continuum from excellent to poor. The social determinants of health can be categorized as distal (e.g. historic, political, social and economic contexts), intermediate (e.g. community infrastructure, resources, systems and capacities), and proximal (e.g. health behaviors, physical and social environment).

The chapter four delves in to the fact about history of self-governance of the Indigenous and how is it influenced by globalization. While there is extensive diversity in Indigenous peoples throughout the world, all Indigenous Peoples have one thing in common—they all share a history of injustice: they have been killed, tortured and enslaved. Through most of North and South America and through much of the Third World has witnessed an overwhelming aggression—legal, physical and psychological—against the Rights of Indigenous Peoples by colonial powers and by other nations. They have been denied the right to participate in governing processes of the current state systems. In many cases, they continue to face threats to their basic existence due to systematic government policies.

The right of self-determination of peoples is a fundamental principle in international law. It is embodied in the Charter of the United Nations and the International Covenant on Civil and Political Rights and the International Covenant on Economic, Social and Cultural Rights. By virtue of that right they freely determine their political status and freely pursue their economic, social and cultural development. The right of self-determination has also been recognized in other international and regional human rights instruments, such as Part VII of the Helsinki Final Act 1975 and Article 20 of the African Charter of Human and Peoples' Rights as well as the Declaration on the Granting of Independence to Colonial Territories and Peoples.

We quote here Mokuau (2011: 98):

> health is that quality of life in which there is an absence of disease, and a presence of general well-being. With holism, all parts of the individual (biological, psychological, social, cognitive, spiritual) and world (individual, family, community, environment) are interconnected.

This is relevant to mention because the majority of these populations has been struggling for their livelihood and their self-determination with limited success; therefore, health issues remain a fact of their lives.

As we discuss the social determinants of health, we note that relatively less literature covers mental health than other health issues. This may be because their other problems are so great that Indigenous mental health issues have received scant attention from researchers. Promoting healthy lives to allow for more community development is of particular importance to communities that are less connected to health-related and socioeconomic infrastructures.

The right of self-determination is central to human rights and broadly acknowledged in the United Nations' Declaration on the Rights of Indigenous People (United Nations, 2007). This means that all Indigenous people, like all other people, possess the right to self-determination, and the right to practice and revitalize cultural traditions and customs. Undoubtedly, the volume of Indigenous health research is increasing; however, change in the health disparities faced by Indigenous peoples when compared with non-Indigenous is slow and insignificant. Walker et al. (2014:3), in support of this, present the example of the gap in life expectancy between Indigenous and non-Indigenous. In their research an interesting and a real comment caught our eyes: "Indigenous researchers and scholars are increasingly challenging traditional Westernized research doctrine." Therefore, a decolonizing approach is important to conduct health research. They further go on to say, quoting (Chilisa, 2012: 14), that the methods of conducting decolonizing research mean that "the worldviews of those who have suffered a long history of oppression and marginalization are given space to communicate from their frames of reference." Consider an example from the United States and the Indigenous there. The United States is home to more than four million Native Americans (Weaver, 2012). More than two-thirds of Native Americans live in urban areas. However, these populations are disproportionately affected by poverty and health disparities.

As we mentioned in previous chapters, being deeply rooted in a land of origin may contribute to an Indigenous identity. Therefore, their cultural identity is intimately connected with their traditional territories, meaning that it is ingrained in the land in a way that they cannot separate from in the event they are displaced (Weaver, 2012). Cultural decay happens when they are removed or displaced and live for a long time away from their traditional land. This means a lot for their health issues. The persistence of Indigenous values underscores their resilience.

Strikingly, the Indigenous youth suicide rates in some North American communities can be 18 times greater than for other young people (Wexler et al., 2014). This in fact reflects their overall status of wellbeing. Lee et al. (2013: 608) reveals that "migrants from Indigenous, pre-Columbian communities in southern Mexico with unique languages and cultural identities comprise a rapidly growing proportion of the U.S. agricultural workforce." In Mexico there are more than 62 distinct ethnolinguistic Indigenous groups with great differences between them, as each preserves their own languages, traditions, and unique ways of life (Linares, 2008). Indigenous Mexicans migrate to the United States with varying levels of identification with a particular minority Indigenous culture, as well as with a majority, mestizo culture.

In many countries, Indigenous populations are distinct from their mainstream populations. Jacobs and Saus (2012) gave in this regard examples of the United States and Norway where there was a boarding-school history followed by a period of child removal, and each of these periods represents negligence and shifting child welfare policies. We have attempted to show that being a developed nation does not necessarily mean that Indigenous rights are protected. For example, according to McDonald (2013) Australia is not a fair country for the Indigenous population. Without doubt Australia is a wealthy country that prioritizes economic over social goals.

> Indigenous Australians live in both relative and absolute poverty, unable to access a decent standard of living and, in many instances, necessities such as food, water, and shelter. The rate of homelessness for Aboriginal and Torres Strait Islanders is four times that of non-Indigenous Australians. The rate of home ownership for Indigenous households is about one-third, compared to two-thirds for non-Indigenous households.
>
> (McDonald, 2013: 4)

A near permanent damage done to the Indigenous peoples, through policies resulting in the forced removal of children from Aboriginal and Torres Strait Islander Families for over 100 years, between 1869 and the 1970s, and other acts of racism, is demonstrated in a swathe of statistics such as decreased life expectancy and low income levels of Aboriginal people (Stewart and Allan, 2013). The Indigenous peoples of Northern Scandinavia and North West Russia are the Saamis, who do not share a common land, but in their own languages they generally refer to their regions as Sa'pmi. "They are not organised into tribes nor are they enrolled in tribal communities. Thus they are solely considered citizens of their respective nations. The four native countries have differing laws regarding Sa'mi, differing legal definitions of 'Sa'miness' and differing Sa'mi self-determination. Generations of harsh assimilation practices and the natural social processes of intermarriage with non-Sa'mi Norwegians have made it difficult to separate out Sa'mis from other Norwegians" (Mary and Merete, 2012: 272).

Globalization has disproportionately impacted Indigenous peoples worldwide, especially in some countries in the South. Therefore, the global efforts in poverty reduction have not witnessed equitable change in poverty measures. Socioeconomic status measures are the current income level, recent income change, poverty flags, current earnings, multi-period averaged incomes and relative position in the income distribution. Empirical studies demonstrate an association between income and morbidity, using various measures of both income and health. Therefore, globalization creates challenges for the global health governance. Since the mid-nineteenth century, globalization of public health has led to the development of international health diplomacy and international regimes for public health. Some characterizations of globalization are, for instance, electronic media, which now reaches families in the remotest rural areas. For example, from Brazilian music in Tokyo to African films in Bangkok, to Shakespeare in Croatia, to books on the history of the Arab world in Moscow, to the CNN world news in Amman, people revel in diversity of the age of globalization (Anyanwu, 2003). The question is how issues of Indigenousness and their health have been affected by globalization.

Historically, approximately 400 million Indigenous people, spanning 70 countries worldwide, have often been dispossessed of their lands, or been in the center of conflict for access to valuable resources because of where they live, or, in yet other cases, are struggling to live the way they would like. Indeed, Indigenous people are often amongst the most disadvantaged people in the world (Shah, 2006). In this globalizing world, there is a wide gap between Indigenous and non-Indigenous peoples by all reckonings of health outcomes and economic empowerment. This gap is even wider in the South. The gap in life expectancy between Indigenous and non-Indigenous population worldwide is alarming. It is nonetheless important to recognize the substantial narrowing of the gap in health between Indigenous and non-Indigenous.

A large proportion of chronic disease in populations could be avoided through primary, secondary, or tertiary services. Avoidable death rates among the Maori, for example, are estimated to be almost double those of Europeans or other New

Zealanders (Tse et al., 2005). Many organizations, however, have been commissioning a number of projects for Indigenous health. An Inter-Agency Support Group (IASG) was established to support the mandate of the Permanent Forum on Indigenous Issues within the United Nations System. In the past five years, the International Labour Organization (ILO), the World Bank, the World Intellectual Property Organization (WIPO), the United Nations Development Programme (UNDP) and the United Nations Children's Fund (UNICEF) have all chaired the IASG. The International Fund currently chairs the group for Agricultural Development (IFAD). In 1982, the Working Group on Indigenous Populations (WGIP) of the Sub-Commission on the Promotion and Protection of Human Rights was established by a decision of the United Nations Economic and Social Council (UN, 2006).

Indigenous people and their communities represent a significant percentage of the global population. They have developed over many generations a holistic traditional scientific knowledge of their lands, natural resources and environment. They enjoy the full measure of human rights and fundamental freedoms without hindrance or discrimination. In view of the interrelationship between the natural environment and its sustainable development and the cultural, social, economic and physical wellbeing of Indigenous people, national and international efforts to implement environmentally sound and sustainable development should recognize, accommodate, promote and strengthen the role of Indigenous people and their communities. Health, a resource for everyday living, is the ability to realize hopes, satisfy needs, change or cope with life experiences, and participate fully in society. Health has physical, mental, social and spiritual dimensions (Sheridan, 2001). Health is influenced by important factors such as the physical environment, health practices and coping skills, biology, health care service and the social and economic environment (the social conditions, or the social determinants of health) in which people live their daily lives (Sheridan, 2001).

The Indigenous community is concrete examples of sustainable societies, historically evolved in diverse ecosystems. Today, they face the challenges of survival and renewal in a globalized world. With the increase in concerns and awareness about the recent global development, Indigenous people want economic development. However, this has indeed caused conflicts with environmental groups when Indigenous people have been given title to land and then proceed to develop just like non-Indigenous people (Xanthaki, 2002). Both historically and in the contemporary world, it is generally the case that states dominate Indigenous people, therefore either displacing them or integrating them into the state (Kunitz, 2000: 1531). Though Norway has constitutionally recognized the Saami as an Indigenous people, their right to Self-Determination according to Article 1 of the UN Covenants on Civil and Political Rights and Economical, Social and Cultural Rights is, however, not yet fully acknowledged by Norway. The Saami Parliament is an Indigenous electoral body (elected every four year) represents the Saami people in all matters concerning them (Sara, 2006).

If trade liberalization as a consequence of globalization is detrimental to economic growth in developing countries, then the current trajectory of the global economy would lead to growing inequalities between advanced and developing countries rather than an eventual convergence (ILO, 2001). The issue of trade liberalization and employment forms part of a broader array of relationships between globalization and labor, including questions of trade and labor standards, social protection, and the role of social dialogue (ILO, 2001). It is also closely related to the liberalization of policies towards foreign direct investment and the role of multinational enterprises (ILO, 2001).

Due to the globalizing force, the government signed the treaty with the PCSJJ in Chittagong Hill Tracts, which led them to self-government, albeit in limited extent. International, bilateral organizations came forward with huge funding for the health improvements of the Indigenous community in the Chittagong area in Bangladesh after the treaty was signed. Now they enjoy access to health services. To overcome poverty, Indigenous people need special assistance that is based on their own objectives and that addresses the barriers they face and helps them protect their livelihoods, heritage and cultural identity. One of the most effective ways of enabling Indigenous people to overcome poverty is to support their efforts to shape and direct their own destinies, and to seek their free, prior and informed consent. Despite the odds, the past decade has seen a notable increase in attention to the concerns of Indigenous people worldwide. One example is that the United Nations proclaimed the opening of the International Decade of the World's Indigenous people on 10 December 1994 (Hall Patrinos, 2004).

Creating market links between Indigenous communities and external buyers can increase incomes and reduce poverty levels. National and local economies can greatly benefit from the contributions of Indigenous people to ecotourism and environmental services (Craib et al., 2003). Among academics, political leaders, and government representatives, differences of opinion and concern abound: differences about the most beneficial structure of self-government, about who controls what, about when self-government should be implemented, about whether or not true form self-government can ever be achieved.

This volume examined how environmental, social, economic, cultural and historical factors influence and determine the social and emotional wellbeing of Aboriginal people, and all indicators showed that Indigenous people are significantly poorer than non-Indigenous people and this reflects on their health. Aboriginal people of all ages carry a heavy burden of illness. The social determinants play a major role in disadvantaging Aboriginal people, and these include colonial history.

Data presented in the papers clearly demonstrates the burdensome health disparities facing all Aboriginal peoples. The evidence is clear that social determinants at proximal, intermediate and distal levels influence health in complex and dynamic ways. The individual and cumulative effects of inequitable social determinants of health are evident in diminished physical, mental, and emotional health experienced by many Aboriginal peoples. Unfavorable distal, intermediate and proximal determinants of health are associated with increased stress through lack of control, diminished immunity and resiliency to disease and social problems, as well as decreased capacity to address ill health. The complex interaction between various determinants appears to create a trajectory of health for individuals that must be addressed through a social determinants approach.

The social, political and economic consequences of being an Indigenous person in Australia, Canada, and New Zealand are significantly affecting the health and wellbeing of the Indigenous people of those countries. Solutions are not easy, but the current situation is not acceptable. For substantial and long-lasting changes to be made, a long-term commitment throughout the community and government sectors is also required. The struggle is not over. The Indigenous peoples, through their cooperation as a group against a system that was slowly crushing them and erasing their identities, have gone international and stabilized their rights in international, national, and even local agreements between their governments, in order to regain their legitimate rights, according to their ancestral history, over the use of their territories. What was really impressive is how they played with the same tools and by the same rules to win one of the most important battles for their existence and wellbeing. The battle has not finished yet, but at least now they know that it is possible to resist and earn real gains that will enable them to better govern their lands according to their cultures and what they believe in. Many of the writers on this topic agree that the Indigenous peoples have been able to stand up for their beliefs and not follow the lead of the dominant societies and governments where they live and that they resist. Also, most of the literature, such as (Martinez, 2012), agrees that the fight over the autonomy of the Indigenous peoples' ancestral lands is not just economic and political, but it is cultural as well.

We got introduced to Indigenous peoples' culture throughout this struggle. I think it is useful now that the whole world know how important the territories that they inhibit are because of the historical value that they carry. Consequently, even if governments wanted to compensate them with another lands in order to make way for their use of the natural resources for the greater benefit of the public, as they portray it, it is enough for them. And it is crucial for their wellbeing, as well as for the ecological system, that Mother Earth's resources should not be exploited the way states so often do in order to build their economies. The forces of globalization have reached the many countries inhibited by Indigenous peoples of Latin America. They brought the same changes and the same problems:— environmental, cultural and economic degradation—and Indigenous historical identity was at stake. This time, the conflict for the Indigenous was different from any other conflict that they had undertaken in their history because they were fighting ideas that contradicted their beliefs and disvalued their ancestral culture.

Moreover, Indigenous women have been the most affected because of globalization; the massive industry and productivity that the globalized economy requires totally ignores her role, which is well established in her tribe. Even when jobs are offered as a result of agreements, they target men and leave no opportunity for women, as in the case of Mayan women of Chiapas (Kukokkanen, 2008). The main goal behind these numerous free trade agreements is merely economic; that is why they oppose everything that these Indigenous peoples represent. The Indigenous peoples do not need to follow the footsteps of the West in order to be able to govern themselves and to win complete autonomy over their ancestral lands.

According to the ruling of the International Court of Justice in 1975: "Indigenous governments do not have to emulate European governmental structures to have sovereignty over their territory" (Venne, 1998: 46).

The homogenous product of the new globalized system, which aims to produce an identical western pattern to be applied for the whole world, a system that does not embrace or understand the culture of diversity and authenticity like the cultures of the Indigenous peoples. It requires them to let go of their beliefs in order to fit into the new liberal market model with a sole focus on economic development, disregarding the culture and environmental aspects. The struggle has arisen throughout Latin American countries, but I agree with Brian Cesarotti (2000) when he said that the outcomes differed from one country to another; for example, Bolivia was able to elect an Indigenous president because of the Indigenous people's majority in the country and pressure the state system for political participation through massive protests, which was able to defeat the outside forces and make a clear path for Indigenous development. Mexico, due to its proximity to the USA, was less able to do so, and also because of the Indigenous populations' minority status (Cesarotti 2005). Now, the Latin American governments are encountering resistance from their Indigenous populations, who demand their collective rights to self-governance on their territories. It has been demonstrated before that they were able to enshrine some of these laws in the national legislations and international agreements and treaties; however, it is very important to implement them on the ground (Martinez, 2008).

Much of the first part of chapter 2 is devoted to forming a definition of the object population of the research—IPs—but definitions are brought forward, then set aside, as being too general or too specific, until the reader has no real understanding of exactly who is being talked about. The final, accepted definition is so wide—as all the world's great variety of IPs are attempted to be included—that its form, in the end ("inhabiting their own historical territory," "having their own historical customs, dress and way of life," "having been colonized by a stronger power," etc.) even when taken together, means that the Mayans were IPs compared to the Aztecs.

There are many concrete additional descriptors of IPs—historically dependent on what are now considered outmoded "un-modern" or archaic means of securing their existence. In the aggregate, they are male dominated societies; beliefs that, no matter how traditional, in a scientific epoch (filled with satellites that look down upon them) have been long ago superseded by experimentally verifiable understandings; in contemporary political default understandings, IPs do not themselves have any understanding of "rights," much less universally applicable declarations of the same (although the dominant hegemony has agencies that apply such notions to them); they have loyalties first to their ethnicity, and secondarily to a modern state; etc.

Health is restricted to infant mortality, longevity, deaths from disease, etc.—what we normally associate with WHO. But WHO itself, in a classic case of "mission creep," has come to define health as the universe of all those things that are related, in any way, to the physical (and because the emotions and mind are lodged in the body, by extension the psychological) wellbeing of an individual or people. This definition is deployed throughout the book, episodically. And so we have actually two definitions: one that is so restricted that only a restricted class of SDHs apply to it directly, and another that is so broad that everything remotely related to social behavior is a valid SDH.

Globalization—the standard understanding of globalization as an economic hegemony of the neoliberal will to power—is used throughout. Yet, although the book is critical of the neoliberal program, it, like neoliberalism, restricts its criticism to political economy: the political outcomes of the economic/trade hegemony and its sole focus on profit and any political arrangement that furthers this.

The world is, in fact, shrinking, quite apart from trade connections and integration. The Tuareg have mobiles; some of the tribal villages of Nepal have direct satellite uplinks; the Amerindians of Suriname watch satellite TV powered by diesel generators; the Saramacca have outboards; etc. There is a way in which no ethnic group is any longer "isolated" in its territory, if the word "territory" means not just land, but the frontiers of a known world that contained the ethnicity/tribe/people. This phenomenon, which we might call anthropological globalization, rather than trade globalization, is a very real phenomenon which is related to the neoliberal program but is not only much more universal than it, but reaches farther back into history, certainly since what is euphemistically called the "age of discovery," most likely even farther back. What does this make of the identification of a "unique people with their own unique culture in their own unique territory"?

The whole notion of rights has deep roots in Western notions of the individual—whatever the UNDRIP and similar documents attempt to set down, by law only individuals have, and can exercise, a right—and its application legally to groups is complicated and problematic for Western law.

Moreover, being a distinctly Western notion firmly embedded in Western (European and Greco-Roman) culture, it is in fact, for IPs, one of the colonial concepts they would reject; unless of course it would be a case of turning the conquerors' own notions against them to get rid of them. But this still fails to confront the problem of what becomes of rights—say the rights of women or children—in a self-governing IP entity.

There is a paradox of what the research thinks IPs would like. On the one hand, there is strong and passionate advocacy for self-determination for IPs to become autochthonous agents of their own endogenous development, the latter meaning the future course of their lives as they see fit. This would, most importantly, include their ability to preserve their own culture, way of life, livelihoods, customs, social institutions, etc.

On the other hand, there is a passionate implied rebuke to the development community for the social exclusion from the "modernity project" of the IPs. Indeed, this is the whole point of many of the statistics cited. According to this point of view, it is the lack of participation in the modernity project, especially within developing nations, that is the miserable destiny of the world's IPs. Social exclusion is the most important factor in the health (narrowly or broadly defined) of IPs.

But, these two points of view are not an easy analytical fit, although they are easy enough to put together in the book. The whole notion of the modernity project—modernization and its later variant, neoliberalism—is a Western project and cultural construction, filled with the default understandings, tacit assumptions, and affective associations of the hegemonic culture of the West, not to mention its ways of ordering things politically, economically, socially, culturally and psychologically. It is to argue for IP inclusion into the very world that is the reason for the undermining of their way of life.

Modern nation-states are jealous of their sovereignty, which is measured in very real terms not in the vaguer categories of culture. Does self-determination include defense? Trade treaties? Foreign policy? Foot dragging by states, something constantly criticized in the book, is quite understandable given the lack of specification of exactly what self-determination encompasses, since all has simply been cast not in the discourse of realpolitik but in the discourse of "rights."

A strong state exhorts the population within its borders to citizenship, primary loyalty to the state (government as representing the nation), contributing revenue to run the state, patriotism, etc. IP actions for self-determination will be looked upon as disloyal, uncitizenlike, tax dodging, etc. to a strong state. A weak state, on the other hand, cannot be depended upon to protect IP resources or territory (through national policing or defense forces), nor can it protect IPs from unfair arrangements with transnational corporations. A weak state also provides weak revenues for already established compensation or claims. So, in either case, the national state is problematic for IP aspirations. The complexity and trade-offs of this problem must be explored in some detail if we are to make sense of the aspirations of IPs to self-determination and self-governance with a view to improving their SDHs, and therefore their health. So further research could be conducted to explore them.

The importance of this problematic can be appreciated if we compare IP aspirations to self-governance with regional aspirations to self-governance. Many of the latter, such as Catalonia in Spain, have their own language and customs, particular history which flows into the present intact, and have inhabited for centuries a very well defined territory. But no one would call the Catalans an IP; yet they have many of the same problems of attempting self-governance within an already existing sovereign state with a Constitution as an IP would.

Diversity—if one half of the argument in the book (and for most development researchers, I might add) is for IPs not to be socially excluded from the modernization or modernity project of the West, or what passes for the latter in developing societies, then such an argument also commits IPs to some form of assimilation into the culture of modernity (material and personal choice, individualism, consumerism, etc.).

To this extent, as has happened the world over (and thus provoking ethical reactions that are deeply ambivalent and ambiguous), the modernity project of development is a form of cultural mono-cropping: there is really only one form that modern progress takes leading to prosperity and development (this includes its culture, even if this is denied by neoliberals). As IPs are assimilated into development, their own culture, as a real existing way of life, begins to fade, more or less depending upon the degree of assimilation.

This raises the question about why the absolute value of diversity is trumpeted whenever the discussion of Indigenous peoples arises. We know about the absolute value of genetic diversity to the adaptive ability of species (that's what sex is all about), but what about sociocultural diversity? What value does it have? I have confronted this many times—there are many who see modernization as the successive convergence of all cultures, so that IPs are merely those modern individuals that are so much like the rest of us except they wear weird clothes and have some strange customs, but are basically rational, self-interested consuming individuals—and have developed arguments for the absolute value of diversity which are interesting.

References

Aboriginal Affairs and Northern Development Canada. 11 June 2008. *Prime Minister Harper Offers Statement of Apology on Behalf of Canadians for the Indian Residential Schools System*. Ottawa. Available online at: http://www.aadnc-aandc.gc.ca/eng/1100100015644/1100100015649 [Accessed on 12 May 2013].

Aboriginal Women's Health and Healing Research Group. 2005. *Annotated Bibliography of Aboriginal Women's Health and Healing Research*. Vancouver, British Columbia: University of British Columbia.

Achim, S., and Gonzalo, O. 2004. Indigenous Knowledge and Natural Resource Management: Local Pathways to Global Development. World Bank Report. Washington, DC: World Bank.

Achim, V. 1998. *The Roma in Romanian History*. Budapest, Hungary: Central European University Share Company.

Adelson, N. 2005. The embodiment of inequality: Health disparities in Aboriginal Canada. *Canadian Journal of Public Health* 96(2): 545–561.

African Commission on Human and Peoples' Rights, University of Pretoria Center for Human Rights and International Labour Organization. 2009. *The Constitutional and Legislative Protection of the Rights of Indigenous Peoples: Eritrea*. The European Commission & DANIDA.

Agrawal, N., André, R., Berger, R., Escarfuller, W., and Sabatini, C. 2012. *Political Representation & Social Inclusion: A Comparative Study of Bolivia, Colombia, Ecuador, and Guatemala*. New York: The Americas Society.

AIPP. 2007. *Annual Report 2007*. Chiangmai: AIPP Foundation.

Ajunnginiq Centre. 2008. *Sexual Health: Resources for Inuit and Aboriginal Peoples in Canada*. Ottawa, Ontario: National Aboriginal Health Organization.

Alan, J., Burmas, M., Preen, D., and Pfaff, J. 2011. Inpatient hospital use in the first year after release from prison: A Western Australian population-based record linkage study. *Australian & New Zealand Journal of Public Health* 35: 265–269. doi: 10.1111/j.1753-6405.2011.00704.x.

Alba, F. 1977. *La Poblacio Un de Mexico: Elucion Dilemas*. Mexico City: El Colegio de Mexico.

Alberta Government. 1984. *Response to Case Management Review Northwest Region*. Report on Richard Cardinal Case. Edmonton: Department of Social Services and Community Health.

Alfaro, L. 2004. Capital controls: A political economy approach. *Review of International Economics* 12(4): 571-590.

Alfred, G.T. 2009. Colonialism and state dependency. *Journal of Aboriginal Health* 5(2): 42–60.

Altman J., Biddle, N., Boyd. H. 2008. The challenge of 'closing the gaps' in Indigenous socioeconomic outcomes. *CAEPR* Topical Issue No. 8/2008. Centre for Aboriginal Economic Policy Research. Australia: Australian National University.

AMAP. 1997. *Arctic Pollution Issues: A State of the Arctic Environment Report.* Oslo, Norway: Arctic Monitoring and Assessment Programme.

AMAP. 1998. *AMAP Assessment Report: Arctic Pollution Issues.* Oslo, Norway: Arctic Monitoring and Assessment Programme.

Aminuzzaman, S.M., and Monjurul Kabir, A.H. 2005. *Role of Parliament in Conflict Resolution: A Critical Review of the Chittagong Hill Tract (CHT) Peace Accord in Bangladesh.* Working Paper No. 2. The Role of Parliament in Conflict and Post Conflict Asia, United Nations Development Programme (UNDP), Regional Centre in Bangkok, Thailand, p. 8.

Anaya, J. 1996. *Indigenous Peoples in International Law.* Oxford: Oxford University Press.

The Anchorage Declaration. 24 April 2009. *Anchorage Declaration.* Available online at: http://unfccc.int/resource/docs/2009/smsn/ngo/168.pdf

Anderson, A.B., and Frideres, J.S. 1981. *Ethnicity in Canada: Theoretical Perspectives.* Toronto: Butterworth and Co.

Anderson, I., Baum, F., and Bentley, M. (Eds.). 2007. *Beyond Bandaids: Exploring the Underlying Social Determinants of Aboriginal Health.* Darwin, Australia: Cooperative Research Centre for Aboriginal Health.

Anderson, M., Smylie, J., Anderson, I., Sinclair, R., and Crengle, S. 2006. *First Nations, Métis and Inuit Health Indicators in Canada. A Background Paper for the Project: Action Oriented Indicators of Health and Health Systems Development for Indigenous Peoples in Australia, Canada and New Zealand.* Melbourne: University of Melbourne.

Anyanwu, A. March 2003. The health of Indigenous people depends on genetics, politics, and socioeconomic factors. *British Medical Journal* 326(7388): pp. 510–511.

Arizpe, L. 2005. Culture, governance and globalization. *Development* 48(1): 35–39.

Armitage, A. 1999. Comparing Aboriginal policies: The colonial legacy. In J. Hylton (ed.), *Aboriginal Self-Government in Canada.* Saskatoon, Canada: Purich Publishing, pp. 61–77.

Asch, M. 1992. Aboriginal self-government and the construction of Canadian constitutional identity. *Alberta Law Review* 30: 465.

Asian Centre for Human Rights (ACHR) 2004. The ravaged hills of Bangladesh, ACHR Review, Index: Review/35/2004. Available at http://www.achrweb.org/Review/2004/35-04:html [Accessed 20 July 2015].

Asian Development Bank. 2002. *Indigenous Peoples/Ethnic Minorities and Poverty Reduction. Regional Report.* Manila: Asian Development Bank.

Assembly of First Nations. 1994. *First Nations Health Commission Annual Report 1993–94.* Ottawa, Ontario: Assembly of First Nations.

Atkin, W.R. 1988–89. *Understanding the Health Care System and Its Impact on First Nations Child & Family Services. Child & Family Services Program Centre on Policy and Research with Respect to First Nations Child & Family Services of Northern Manitoba.* Thompson: Awasis Child & Family Services.

Atkinson, D.L. 2008. *Aboriginal Health Promotion: A Literature Review and Environmental Scan.* Vancouver: BC Initiatives for Aboriginal Health, pp. 1–55.

Auger, N., Raynault, M.F., Lessard, R., and Choinière, R. 2004. Income and health in Canada. In D. Raphael (ed.), *Social Determinants of Health.* Toronto: Canadian Scholars' Press Inc., pp. 21–38.

Australian Bureau of Statistics (ABS). 2002. *Housing and Infrastructure in Aboriginal and Torres Strait Islander Communities*. [Cat. No. 4710.0]. Canberra: Australian Bureau of Statistics.

Australian Bureau of Statistics (ABS). 2003. *The Health and Welfare of Australia's Aboriginal and Torres Strait Islander Peoples*. [Cat. No. 4704.0]. Canberra: Australian Bureau of Statistics.

Australian Bureau of Statistics (ABS). 2004. *National Aboriginal and Torres Strait Islander Social Survey 2002*. [Cat. No. 4714.0]. Canberra: Australian Government Publishing Service.

Australian Bureau of Statistics (ABS). 2005. *The Health and Welfare of Australia's Aboriginal and Torres Strait Islander Peoples*. [Cat. No. 4704.0]. Canberra: Australian Bureau of Statistics.

Australian Bureau of Statistics (ABS). 2010. *Aboriginal and Torres Strait Islander Suicide Deaths*. Canberra: Australian Bureau of Statistics.

Australian Health Ministers' Advisory Council. 2011. *Aboriginal and Torres Strait Islander Health Performance Framework Report 2010*. Canberra: AHMAC.

Australian Institute of Health and Welfare and Australian Bureau of Statistics. 2005. *The Health and Welfare of Australia's Aboriginal and Torres Strait Islander Peoples 2005*. [ABS Cat. No. 4704.0]. Canberra: Commonwealth of Australia, p. 148.

Australians for Native Title & Reconciliation (ANTaR). 2007. *Success Stories in Indigenous Health: A Showcase of Successful Aboriginal and Torres Strait Islander Health Projects*. Sydney: ANTaR.

Aylwin, J. 2006. Land policy and Indigenous peoples in Chile: Progress and contradictions in a context of economic globalization. Paper presented at Land, Poverty, Social Justice & Development International Conference, Institute of Social Studies, The Hague, Netherlands, January, 9–14.

Bambas, A., Casas, J.A., Drayton, H.A., and Valdés, A. (Eds.) 2000. *Health and Human Development in the New Global Economy: The Contributions and Perspectives of Civil Society in the Americas*. Washington, DC: Pan American Health Organization (PAHO/WHO).

Barker, D. 2007. The Rise and Predictable Fall of Globalized Industrial Agriculture. San Francisco: International Forum on Globalization (IFG).

Barras, B., Blaser, M., Feit, HA., and McRae, G. 2004. Life projects: Development our way. In *The Way of Development: Indigenous Peoples, Life Projects and Globalization*. Ottawa: IDRC.

Baskin, C. 2007. Circles of resistance: Spirituality and transformative change in social work education and practice. In J. Coates, J.R. Graham, B. Swartzentruber, and B. Ouelette (eds.), *Spirituality and social work: Selected Canadian readings*. Toronto: Canadian Scholars' Press Inc., pp. 191–211.

BBC. 26 May 2006. Indigenous people 'worst-off world over'. Available online at: http://news.bbc.co.uk/2/hi/europe/5019582.stm#graph [Accessed on 29 June 2010].

BBC. 11 April 2016. Canadian Attawapiskat First Nation suicide emergency. Available online at: http://www.bbc.com/news/world-us-canada-36012578

Beatty, B.B., and Berdahl, L. 2011. Health care and Aboriginal seniors in urban Canada: Helping a neglected class. *The International Indigenous Policy Journal* 2(1):1–16.

Bell, C.E. 1993. Comment on 'partners in confederation': A report on self-government by the Royal Commission on Aboriginal peoples. *U.B.C. Law Review* 27: 361.

Bell, C.E. 1999. Métis self-government: The Alberta Settlement Model. In John H. Hylton (ed.), *Aboriginal Self-Government in Canada: Current Trends and Issues*, 2nd edn. Saskatoon: Purich Publishing, pp. 329–351.

Bern, J., and Dodds, S. 2000. On the plurality of interests: Aboriginal self-government and land rights. In D. Ivison, P. Patten and W. Sanders (eds.), *Political Theory and the Rights of Indigenous Peoples*. Cambridge, UK: Cambridge University Press, pp. 163–182.

Bird, M.E. September 2002. Health and Indigenous people: Recommendations for the next generation. *American Journal of Public Health* 92(9):1391–1392.

Blaser, M., Feit, H.A., and McRae, G. (Eds.). 2008. *In Way of Development: Indigenous Peoples, Life Projects and Globalization*. London: Zed Books.

Blust, R. 1999. Subgrouping, circularity and extinction: Some issues in Austronesian comparative linguistics. In E. Zeitoun and P.J.K. Li (eds.), *Selected Papers from the Eighth International Conference on Austronesian Linguistics*. Taipei: Academia Sinica, pp. 31–94.

Borrows, J.J. 1997. Wampum at Niagara: The Royal Proclamation, Canadian legal history, and self-government. In Michael Asch (ed.), *Aboriginal and Treaty Rights in Canada: Essays on Law, Equality, and Respect for Difference*. Vancouver: UBC Press, pp. 155–173.

Bowen, J.R. August 2000. Should we have a universal concept of 'Indigenous peoples' rights'?: Ethnicity and essentialism in the twenty-first century. *Anthropology Today* 16(4): 12–16.

Brady, M. 1984. Contradictions and consequences: The social and health status of Canada's registered Indian population. In J. Fry (ed.), *Contradictions in Canadian Society: Readings in Introductory Sociology*. Toronto: Wiley & Sons, pp. 140–155.

Brant, C.C. 1990. Native ethics and rules of behaviour. *Canadian Journal of Psychiatry* 35: 534–539.

British Columbia. June 2002. *The Health & Well-Being of Aboriginal Children and Youth in British Columbia*. British Columbia: Ministry of Children and Family Development. Available online at: www.gov.bc.ca/mcf

Brosius, J.P. 1999. Analyses and interventions: Anthropological engagements with environmentalism. *Current Anthropology* 40: 277–309.

Brown, R. 2001. Australian Indigenous mental health. *Australian and New Zealand Journal of Mental Health Nursing* 10(1): 33–41.

Burger, J. 1987. *Report From the Frontier: The State of the World's Indigenous Peoples*. London: Zed Books.

Callister, P., Didham, R., and Kivi, A. 2009. Who are we? The conceptualisation and expression of ethnicity. *Official Statistics Research Series*, 4 Wellington: Statistics New Zealand. Vol 4: 5–45.

Canada. 1990. *First Nations Mental Health Summary Report: Proceedings of Thematic Focus Group Meetings Held during 1989–90*. Ottawa: Health and Welfare Canada, Medical Services Branch, Indian and Northern Health Services, Mental Health Advisory Services.

Canadian Diabetes Association. 2004. *The Prevalence and Costs of Diabetes*. Available online at: www.diabetes.ca/ Section_about/prevalence.asp

Canadian Institute for Health Information. 1999. *Statistical Report on the Health of Canadians*. Prepared by the Federal, Provincial and Territorial Advisory Committee on Population Health for the Meeting of Ministers of Health, Charlottetown, P.E.I., September 16–17.

Canadian Institute for Health Information. 2000. *Health Care in Canada 2000: A First Annual Report (Brochure)*. Available online at: http://www.cihi.ca/Roadmap/Health_ Rep/healthreport2000/pdf/eng-brochure.pdf [Accessed on 23 March 2012].

Canadian Institute for Health Research. 2007. *CIHR Guidelines for Health Research Involving Aboriginal People*. Ottawa, Ontario: Canadian Institute of Health Research, pp. 1–46.

Canadian Institute of Child Health. 2000. *The Health of Canada's Children: A CICH Profile*, 3rd edn. Ottawa, Ontario: Canadian Institute of Child Health.

Canadian Institute of Child Health. 2004. *The Health of Canada's Children: A CICH Profile: Income Inequity*. Available online at: http://www.cich.ca/PDFFiles/ProfileFact Sheets/English/Incomeinequity.pdf [Accessed on 23 June 2008].

Canadian UNICEF Committee. 2009a. *Aboriginal Children's Health: Leaving No Child Behind*. Toronto, Ontario: UNICEF Canada.

Canadian UNICEF Committee. 2009b. Canada's Supplement to the State of the World's Children 2009. *Aboriginal Children's Health: Leaving No Child Behind*. Available online at: http://www.itk.ca/sites/default/files/Leaving_no_child_behind_09.pdf [Accessed on 18 October 2011].

Cariño, J. April 2005. Indigenous peoples, human rights and poverty. *Indigenous Perspectives* 7(1): 28–46.

Carson, B., Dunbar, T., Chenhall, R., and Bailie, R. 2007. *Social Determinants of Indigenous Health*. Australia: Allen & Unwin.

Castles, S. 1998. Globalization and migration: Some pressing contradictions. *International Social Science Journal* 50(156):179 – 186.

Castles, S. 2002. Environmental change and forced migration: Making sense of the debate. Refugees Studies Centre. University of Oxford. Working Paper No. 70. October. Oxford: University of Oxford.

CELADE. 1992. Boletin Demografico. No 50. Latin America Census Information about Indigenous people. Santiago de Chile: CELADE.

Cesarotti, B. 2000. Globalization's Impact on Indigenous peoples in Mexico and Bolivia. Grand Valley State University, Michigan.

Chadwick, E. 1965. *Report on the Sanitary Condition of the Labouring Population of Great Britain, 1842*. Edinburgh, UK: Edinburgh University Press.

Chakraborty, E. 2004. Understanding Women's Mobilization in the Chittagong Hill Tracts Struggle: The Case of Mahila Samiti. Paper Presented to the 15th Biennial Conference of the Asian Studies Association of Australia in Canberra, 29 June to 2nd July.

Chandler, M.J., and Lalonde, C.E. 1998. Cultural continuity as a hedge against suicide in Canada's First Nations. *Transcultural Psychiatry* 35: 191–219.

Chapleaucree. 1996. *Recent History-Aboriginal Self Government. Chronology of Events July 1994–June 1998*. Canada: Queens University. Available online at: http://www.global issues.org/HumanRights/Indigenous/ [Accessed on 18 August 2016].

Chartier, C. 1999. Aboriginal self-government and the Métis nation. In John H. Hylton (ed.), *Aboriginal Self-Government in Canada: Current Trends and Issues*, 2nd edn. Saskatoon: Purich Publishing, pp. 112–124.

Chartrand, P.L.A.H. 1993. Aboriginal self-government: The two sides of legitimacy. In Susan D. Phillips (ed.), *How Ottawa Spends, 1993–1994: A More Democratic Canada . . .?*. Ottawa: Carleton University Press, pp. 231–256.

Chhakchhuak, P.S. 2004. *Chittagong Hill Tracts: Stating and Resolving the Issues within the Mountains*. American International School/Dhaka, Senior Project.

Chilisa, B. 2012. *Indigenous Research Methodologies*. London: Sage Publications.

Cholchester, M. 1995. Indigenous peoples' rights and sustainable resource use in South and Southeast Asia. In R.H. Barnes, A. Gray and B. Kingsbury (eds.), *Indigenous Peoples in Asia*. Ann Arbor, MI: Association for Asian Studies, University of Michigan.

Chomsky, N. 2006. *Failed States: The Abuse of Power and the Assault on Democracy*. New York: Metropolitan Books/Henry Holt.

Christensen, M., and Manson, S. 2001. Adult attachment as a framework for understanding mental health and American Indian families: A study of three family cases *American Behavioral Scientist* 44(9): 1447–1465.

Christian, E. 2008. *The Concept of Indigenous Peoples in Asia: A Resource Book.* [IWGIA Document No. 123]. Copenhagen: International Work Group for Indigenous Affairs (IWGIA).

Christie, G. 2002. *Challenges to Urban Aboriginal Governance.* [Unpublished]. Institute of Intergovernmental Relations, Queen's University. Available online at: www.iigr.ca/conferences/archive/pdfs3/Christie.pdf [Accessed on 27 July 2009].

Clark, B. 1990. *Native Liberty, Crown Sovereignty: The Existing Aboriginal Right of Self-Government in Canada.* Montreal: McGill-Queen's University Press.

Clough, A.R., D'Abbs, P., Cairney, S., Gray, D., Maruff, P., Parker, R., and O'Reilly, B. 2005. Adverse mental health effects of cannabis use in two Indigenous communities in Arnhem Land, Northern Territory, Australia: Exploratory study. *Australian and New Zealand Journal of Psychiatry* 39: 612–620.

Cole, M. 2003. Youth sexual health in Nunavut: A needs based survey of knowledge, attitudes and behaviour. *International Journal of Circumpolar Health* 63: 270–273.

Collier, G., and Collier, J. July 2005. The Zapatista rebellion in the context of globalization. *Journal of Peasant Studies* 32(3/4): 450–460. doi:10.1080/03066150500266794 [Accessed on 18 January 2014].

Cooney, P. 2006. *The Decline of Neoliberalism and the Role of Social Movements in Latin America.* Paper presented at the X Jornadas de Economía Crítica, Alternativas al capitalismo, Barcelona, Spain, March 23–25.

Cornell, S., and Kalt, J.P. 2003. *Alaska Native Self-Government and Service Delivery: What works?* Joint Occasional Papers on Native Affairs, No. 2003–01. Cambridge, MA: HPAIED.

Country Health Information Profiles. 2010. *Papua New Guinea.* Available online at: http://www.wpro.who.int/countries/png/25PNGpro2011_finaldraft.pdf [Accessed on 10 May 2014].

Craib, K.J.P., Spittal, P.M., Wood, E., Laliberte, N., Hogg, R.S., and Li, K. 2003. Risk factors for elevated HIV incidence among Aboriginal injection drug users in Vancouver. *CMAJ* 168(1):19–24.

Crowe, D.M. 1994. *A History of the Gypsies of Eastern Europe and Russia.* New York, NY: St. Martin's Press.

Crowshoe, C. 2005. *Consulting Inc.* Prepared for the First Nations Centre National Aboriginal Health Organization First Nations Centre (FNC). National Aboriginal Health Organization (NAHO).

Crystal, D. 2000. *Language Death.* Cambridge: Cambridge University Press.

Curry-Stevens, A. 2004. Income and income distribution. In D. Raphael (ed.), *Social Determinants of Health.* Toronto: Canadian Scholars' Press Inc., pp. 21–38.

Curtis, L. 2007. *Health Status of On and Off-Reserve Aboriginal Peoples: Analysis of the Aboriginal Peoples Survey.* Social and Economic Dimensions of an Aging Population Research Papers. Hamilton: McMaster University.

Cyr, J. 2001. Role of community consultation in self-governance. In J. Oakes, R. Riewe, M. Bennett and B. Chisholm (eds.), *Pushing the Margins.* University of Manitoba: Native Studies Press, pp. 196–203.

Czyzewski, K. 2011. Colonialism as a broader social determinant of health. *The International Indigenous Policy Journal* 2(1): 1–14.

Dacks, G. 1986. The case against dividing the Northwest Territories. *Canadian Public Policy* 12(1): 202–213.

David Eller, J. 1997. Ethnicity, culture, and 'the past'. *Michigan Quarterly Review* XXXVI(4): 552–599.

Davies, J.-M., and Mazumder, A. 2003. Health and environmental policy issues in Canada: The role of watershed management in sustaining clean drinking water quality at surface sources. *Journal of Environmental Management* 68: 273–286.

Decade Watch, 2007. Decade watch update. Romania: Decade Watch.

Demographic Bulletin. 1992. *Operationalization of the Term 'Indigenous people' Is a Difficult Task.* United Nation's Latin American Demographic Center. No. 50. Santiago: UNCELADE.

Department of Aboriginal Development. 2012. *Number of Orang Asli Villages and Population by State, 2012.* Available online at: http://www.rurallink.gov.my/c/document_library/get_file?uuid=42c6544e-c38d-45bdabda-2b6501570ab6&groupId=977333 [Accessed on 15 August 2013].

Department of Indian Affairs and Northern Development (DIAND). 1990. *You Wanted to Know: Some Answers to the Most Often Asked Questions about Programs and Services for Registered Indians in Canada.* Report: QS 6141000BBA1. Ottawa: DIAND.

Department of Indian Affairs and Northern Development (DIAND). 1996. *Aboriginal Women: A Demographic, Social and Economic Profile.* Repot. QS3557010BBA1. Ottawa: DIAND.

Deruyttere, A. 2001. *Pueblos indígenas, globalización y desarrollo con identidad: algunas reflexiones de estrategia. Banco Interamericano de Desarrollo.* Available online at: http://www.iadb.org/sds/doc/Ind-ADLasaWP.pdf [Accessed on 18 January 2014].

Dhamai, B.M. 2006. *Migration and Indigenous People: A Perspective of Bangladesh.* Presented in the Expert Workshop on Indigenous Peoples and Migration, Geneva, April 6–7.

Diamond, J.N. 2001. *Why Did Human History Unfold Differently on Different Continents for the Last 13,000 Years?.* Santa Monica, CA: RAND Corporation. Available online at: http://www.rand.org/pubs/papers/P8054 [Accessed on 11 October 2010].

Díaz, H. 1997. *Indigenous Peoples in Latin America: The Quest for Self-Determination.* Boulder, CO: Westview Press.

Dictaan-Bang-oa, E. 2004. *In Search for Peace in the Chittagong Hill Tracts of Bangladesh.* Baguio City, Philippines: Tebtebba (Indigenous Peoples International Centre for Policy Research and Education).

Dinorah, A. 2001. *An Assessment of Democratization and Peace in Guatemala.* Paper delivered at the Congress of the Canadian Association for Latin American and Caribbean Studies (CALACS). Antigua Guatemala. Panel: Peace and Democratization in Guatemala. Paper: An Assessment of Peace and Democracy in Guatemala, 20–21 April, 2001. York University. Canada.

Dion Stout, M. 1997. Family violence in Aboriginal communities. In J. Rick Ponting (ed.), *First Nations in Canada: Perspectives on Opportunity, Empowerment, and Self-Determination.* Toronto: McGraw-Hill Ryerson Limited, pp. 273–298.

Dion Stout, M., and Kipling, G.D. 1999. *Emerging Priorities for the Health of First Nations and Inuit Children and Youth.* Paper prepared for Strategic Policy, Planning and Analysis Directorate, First Nations and Inuit Health Branch (FNIHB). Available online at: www.hc-sc.gc.ca/fnihb/sppa/ppp/emerging_priorities_youth.htm#LiteratureReviewand Analysis [Accessed on 24 September 2009].

Durey, A., and Thompson, S.C. 2012. Reducing the health disparities of Indigenous Australians: Time to change focus. *BMC Health Services Research* 12: 151. doi:10.1186/1472-6963-12-151

Durst, D. 1996a. *First Nations Self-Government of Social Services: An Annotated Bibliography.* Regina: University of Regina, Social Administration Research Unit, Faculty of Social Work, pp. 3–108.

Durst, D. 1996b. The circle of self-government: A guide to Aboriginal government of social services. In R. Delaney, K. Brownlee and M.K. Zapf (eds.), *Issues in Northern*

Social Work Practice. Thunder Bay: Centre for Northern Studies, Lakehead University, pp. 104–124.

Durst, D. 1996c. *The Circle of Self-Government: An Observer's Field Guide to Aboriginal Government of Social Services*. Regina: University of Regina, Social Administration Research Unit, Faculty of Social Work, pp. 5–14.

Durst, D., McDonald, J., and Rich, C. 1993. *Aboriginal Self-Government and Social Services: Finding the Path to Empowerment*. Conne River Reserve, NF: Council of the Conne River Micmacs.

Dwyer, J., Shannon, S., and Godwin, S. 2007. *Learning from Action: Management of Aboriginal and Torres Strait Islander Health Services*. Darwin: Cooperative Research Centre for Aboriginal Health.

Dyck, R., Klomp, H., Tan, L.K., Turnell, R.W. and Boctor, M.A. March 2002. A comparison of rates, risk factors, and outcomes of gestational diabetes between Aboriginal and non-Aboriginal women in the Saskatoon Health District. *Diabetes Care* 25(3): 487–493.

Eastwell, H. Projective and identificatory illness among ex-hunter gatherers: A seven year survey of a remote Australian Aboriginal community. *Psychiatry* 40: 331–343.

Ekstedt, J.W. 1999. International perspectives on Aboriginal self-government. In John H. Hylton (ed.), *Aboriginal Self-Government in Canada: Current Trends and Issues*, 2nd edn. Saskatoon: Purich Publishing, pp. 45–59.

Erni, C. 2008. The concept of Indigenous peoples in Asia: A resource book. IWGIA Document No. 123. Copenhagen: International Work Group for Indigenous Affairs (IWGIA).

Estey, E.A., Kmetic, A.M., and Redding, J.L. 2010. Thinking about Aboriginal KT: Learning from the Network for Aboriginal Health Research British Columbia (NEARBC). *Canadian Journal of Public Health* 101(1): 83–86.

Federation of Saskatchewan Indians. 1983. *Indian Control of Indian Child Welfare: A Report by the Health and Social Development Commission of the Federation of Saskatchewan Indians*. Saskatchewan Federation of Indians. Regina.

Fellegi, I. September 1997. *On Poverty and Low Income*. Statistics Canada. Available online at: http://www.statcan.ca:80/english/research/13F0027XIE/13F0027XIE.htm

Ferreira, M.L. 2013. *Chapter 2: The UN Declaration on the Rights of Indigenous Peoples*. Minnesota, MN: University of Minnesota Press.

Fidler, D.P. 2001. The globalization of public health: The first 100 years of international health diplomacy. *Bulletin of the World Health Organization* 79(9): 842–849.

First Nations Centre. 2006. *An Annotated Bibliography: Cultural Intervention Models in Mental Health*. Ottawa, Ontario: National Aboriginal Health Organization.

First Nations Regional Longitudinal Health Survey (RHS). 2005. *First Nations Regional Longitudinal Health Survey (RHS) 2002/03: Results for Adults, Youth, and Children Living in First Nations Communities*. Ottawa, Canada: First Nations Health Centre.

First Nations, Inuit and Aboriginal Health. 2007. *First Nations and Inuit Health Program Compendium*. Ottawa, Ontario. Available online at: http://www.hc-sc.gc.ca/fniah-spnia/pubs/aborig-autoch/2007_compendium/index-eng.php

Foek, A. 28 December 2005. Coca farmer wins Bolivian election: New President to challenge multinationals. *CorpWatch*. Oakland. Available online at: http://www.corpwatch.org/article.php?id=12989 [Accessed on 20 October 2010].

Foliaki, S., and Pearce, N. August 2003. Changing pattern of ill health for Indigenous people: Control of lifestyle is beyond individuals and depends on social and political factors. *British Medical Journal* 327(23): 406–407.

Fonesca, I. 1995. *Bury Me Standing: The Gypsies and their Journey*. New York, NY: Vintage Books.

Foster George, K. 2012. Foreign investment and Indigenous peoples: Options for promoting equilibrium between economic development and Indigenous rights. *Michigan Journal of International Law* 33(4): 627–691.

Fox, S.I. 2001. *Self-Government in the Circumpolar World.* Scott Polar Research Institute, University of Cambridge. Available online at: www.spri.cam.ac.uk.

Freedman, B. 1994. The space for Aboriginal self-government in British Columbia: The effect of the decision of the British Columbia Court of appeal in Delgamuukw v. British Columbia. *University of British Columbia Law Review* 28: 49.

Freeman, H., Harten, T., Springer, S., Randall, P., Curran, M.A., and Stone, K. 1992. Industrial pollution prevention: A critical review. *Journal of the Air & Waste Management Association* 42(May): 617–656.

Freitas, C.E.C., Kahn, J.R., and Rivas, A.A.F. 2004. Indigenous people and sustainable development in Amazonas. *International Journal of Sustainable Development & World Ecology* 11: 312–325.

Frideres, J.S. 1996. The Royal Commission on Aboriginal peoples: The route to self-government?. *The Canadian Journal of Native Studies* XVI(2): 247.

Friendly, M. 2004. Early childhood education and care. In D. Raphael (ed.), *Social Determinants of Health: Canadian Perspectives.* Toronto: Canadian Scholars' Press Inc., pp. 128–142.

Gabriel, A., and Verba, S. 1989. *The Civic Culture Revisited.* London: Sage Publications.

Galabuzi, G.E. 2004. Social exclusion. In D. Raphael (ed.), *Social Determinants of Health: Canadian Perspectives.* Toronto: Canadian Scholars' Press Inc., pp. 252–268

Gannon, M. 3 July 2014. *Imperiled Amazon Indians Make 1st Contact with Outsiders.* Available online at: LiveScience.com

Garnett, S.T., and Sithole, B. 2007. *Sustainable Northern Landscapes and the Nexus with Indigenous Health: Healthy Country, Healthy People.* Land and Water Australia, Canberra.

Gaviria, A., and Raphael, S. 2001. Schoolbased peer effects and juvenile behavior. *Review of Economics and Statistics* 83(2): 257–268.

Giddens, A. 2000. *Runaway World: How Globalization is Reshaping our Lives.* New York: Routledge.

Gnerre, M. 1990. Indigenous people in Latin America. Working paper 30. International Fund for Agricultural Development. Rome: IFAD.

Godoy, R., and Cardenas, M. 2000. Markets and the health of Indigenous people: A methodological contribution. *Human Organization* 59(1): 117–125.

Gokalp, D. 2007. *Beyond Ethnopolitical Contention: The State, Citizenship and Violence in the 'New' Kurdish Question in Turkey.* Unpublished PhD thesis.: The University of Texas at Austin, Austin, TX.

Gore, D., and Kothari, A. 2012. Social determinants of health in Canada: Are healthy living initiatives there yet? A policy analysis. *International Journal of Equity Health* 11(41): 1–14.

Gotowiec, A., and Beiser, M. 1993. Aboriginal children's mental health: Unique challenges. *Canada's Mental Health* 41: 7–11.

Government of India, 1991. *A Hand Book of Population Statistics- Census of India- 1991.* India: Government of India.

Grace, S.L. 2003. A review of Aboriginal women's physical and mental health status in Ontario. *Canadian Journal of Public Health* 94: 173–175.

Gracey, M., Murray, H., Hitchcock, N.E., Owles, E.N., and Murphy, B.P. 1983. The nutrition of Australian Aboriginal infants and young children. *Nutrition Research* 3: 133–147.

Graham, J. 2007. *Rethinking Self-Government: Developing a More Balanced, Evolutionary Approach.* [Policy Brief No. 29]. Canada: Institute on Governance.

Graham, K.A. 1999. Urban Aboriginal governance in Canada: Paradigms and prospects. In John H. Hylton (ed.), *Aboriginal Self-Government in Canada: Current Trends and Issues*, 2nd edn. Saskatoon: Purich Publishing, pp. 377–396.

Green, J., and Voyageur, C. 1999. Globalization and development at the bottom. In M. Porter and E. Judd (eds.), *Feminists Doing Development: A Practical Critique*. London: Zed Books, pp. 143–155.

Greenwood, M. 2005. Children as citizens of First Nations: Linking Indigenous health to early childhood development. *Paediatrics and Child Health* 10(9): 553–555.

Greenwood, M.L., and Naomi, S. 2012. Social determinants of health and the future well-being of Aboriginal children in Canada. *Pediatric Child Health* 17(Aug-Sept 7): 381–384.

Gurran, N., and Phipps, P. 2003. Reconciling Indigenous and non-Indigenous land management concepts in planning curricula. Refereed paper presented to the Australian and New Zealand Association of Planning Schools (ANZAPS) Conference, Auckland, 26–28 September. ANZAPS. Auckland, NZ.

Hale, C. 2005. Neoliberal multiculturalism: The remaking of cultural rights and racial dominance in Central America. *POLAR: Political and Legal Anthropology Review* 28(1): 10–28.

Hall, G., and Patrinos, H.A. 2004. *Indigenous Peoples, Poverty and Human Development in Latin America: 1994–2004*. Washington, DC: World Bank.

Hall, G., and Patrinos, H.A. 2006. *Indigenous Peoples, Poverty and Human Development in Latin America: 1994–2004*. London: Palgrave Macmillan.

Hall, G., and Patrinos, H.A. 2010. *Indigenous Peoples, Poverty and Development*. Washington: World Bank.

Hanselmann, C. September 2001. *Urban Aboriginal People in Western Canada: Realities and Policies*. Calgary, Alberta, Canada: Canada West Foundation.

Harcourt, W. 2001. Women's health, poverty and globalization. *Development* 44(1): 85–90 (The Society for International Development, Sage Publications).

Harry, D., Howard, S., and Shelton, B.L. May 2000. *Indigenous Peoples, Genes and Genetics: What Indigenous People Should Know about Biocolonialism.* Stanford School of Medicine Center for Biomedical Ethics. Center for Integration of Research on Genetics and Ethics: Indigenous Peoples Council on Biocolonialism.

Hasan, K. 21 February 2016. Lack of government initiatives threaten Indigenous languages. *Dhaka Tribune.*

Healey, G.K., and Meadows, L.M. 2007. Inuit women's health in Nunavut, Canada: A review of the literature. *International Journal of Circumpolar Health* 66: 199–214.

Health Canada. 1999. *Diabetes in Canada: National Statistics and Opportunities for Improved Surveillance, Prevention, and Control.* Diabetes Division, Bureau of Cardio-Respiratory Diseases and Diabetes, Laboratory Centre for Disease Control Health Protection Branch. Ottawa: Minister of Public Works and Government Services Canada.

Health Canada. 2000. *HIV and AIDS among Aboriginal People in Canada.* HIV/AIDS Epi Update. Population and Public Health Branch (PPHB), Bureau of HIV/AIDS, STD and TB. Available online at: http://www.hc-sc.gc.ca/hpb/lcdc/bah/epi/aborig_e.html April.

Health Canada. 2010. *First Nations, Inuit, and Aboriginal Health: Drinking Water and Wastewater.* Available online at: http://www.hc-sc.gc.ca/fniah-spnia/promotion/public-publique/water-eau-eng.php#how_many [Accessed on 12 November 2011].

Health Canada. 2013. *Acting On What We Know: Preventing Youth Suicide in First Nations.* Ottawa: Health Canada.

Healthinfonet. May 2000. Aboriginal and Torres Strait Islander Health Bulletin: An electronic publication from the Australian Indigenous Health. *InfoNet*, Issue 7, ISSN 1329-3362.

Heart and Stroke Foundation. 2003. *The Growing Burden of Heart Disease and Stroke in Canada 2003*. Available online at: http://ww2.heartandstroke.ca/images/English/Heart_Disease_EN.pdf [Accessed on 4 January 2009].

Helin, S. 1993. Beyond the Caregivers: Health and Social Services Policy for the 1990s. *The Path to Healing: Report of the National Round Table on Aboriginal Health and Social Issues*. Royal Commission on Aboriginal Peoples, pp. 158–170.

Hellard, M.E., Sinclair, M.I., Forbes, A.B., and Fairley, C.K. 2001. A randomized, blinded, controlled trial investigating the gastrointestinal health effects of drinking water quality. *Environmental Health Perspectives* 109(8): 773–778.

Helsinki Human Rights Watch. 1990. *Romania: Human Rights Developments*. Available online at: http://www.hrw.org/reports/1990/WR90/HELSINKI.BOU-02.htm#P171_37792

Hogg, P.W., and Turpel, M.E. 1995. Implementing Aboriginal self-government: Constitutional and jurisdictional issues. *Canadian Bar Review* 74(2): 187–224.

Hornburg, A. 1994. Environmentalism, ethnicity and sacred places. *Canadian Review of Sociology and Anthropology* 31(3): 245–267.

Hossain, D.M. 2013. Socio-economic situation of the Indigenous people in the Chittagong Hill Tracts (CHT) of Bangladesh. *Middle East Journal of Business* 8(2): 22–30.

Hu, J. 2009. Differences in health care utilization and satisfaction with health services among ethnic groups on the Thailand-Myanmar border, 2000–2004. *Journal of Public Health and Development* 7(1): 81–96.

Human Resources Development Canada (HRDC). 1998. *The Market Basket Measure: Constructing a New Measure of Poverty. Applied Research Bulletin* 4(2): 1–4.

Human Rights and Equal Opportunity Commission (HREOC). 2003. *A Statistical* Overview *of Aboriginal and Torres Strait Islander Peoples in Australia*. HREOC, Aboriginal and Torres Strait Islander Social Justice. Available online at: www.humanrights.gov.au/sociaLjustice/statisticslindex.html [Accessed 1 March 2004].

Human Rights Watch. 2005. *Suppressing Dissent: Human Rights Abuses and Political Repression in Ethiopia's Oromia Region*. Available online at: http://www.refworld.org/docid/42c3bd090.html [Accessed on 25 July 2010].

Hunter, B.H., and Schwab, R.G. 2003. Practical reconciliation and continuing disadvantage in Indigenous education. *The Drawing Board: An Australian Review of Public Affairs* 4(2): 83–98.

Hutchins, P.W., Hilling, C., and Schulze, D. 1995. The Aboriginal right to self-government and the Canadian Constitution: The ghost in the machine. *University of British Columbia Law Review* 29: 251.

Hye, H.A.1996. *Below the Line: Rural Poverty in Bangladesh*. Dhaka: University Press Limited.

Hylton, J.H. 1997. The case for Aboriginal self-government: A social policy perspective. In J.H. Hylton (ed.), *Aboriginal Self-Government in Canada: Current Trends and Issues*. Saskatoon: Purich Publishing, pp. 34–48.

Smith Rhona, K.M. 1957. *Text and Materials on International Human Rights*. Geneva: ILO.

ILO. November 2001. *Trade Liberalization and Employment*. Working Party on the Social Dimension of Globalization. WP/GB.282/WP/SDG/2. Geneva: ILO.

ILO. 2008. Key Principles in Implementing ILO Convention No. 169. Geneva: ILO.

ILO and ACHPR. 2009. Overview repot of the research project by the ILO and African Commission on Human and People's Right on the constitutional and legislative protection of the rights of Indigenous peoples in 24 African countries. Geneva: ILO.

Inter-Agency Support Group on Indigenous Peoples' Issues (IASG). 2014. *The Health of Indigenous Peoples*. Thematic Paper Towards the Preparation of the 2014 World Conference on Indigenous Peoples. Available online at: http://www.un.org/en/ga/president/68/pdf/wcip/IASG_Thematic%20paper_Health.pdf

International Fund for Agricultural Development (IFAD). 2002a. *Strategic Framework for IFAD 2002–2006*. Rome: IFAD.

International Fund for Agricultural Development (IFAD). 2002b. *Assessment of Rural Poverty: Latin America and the Caribbean*. Rome: IFAD.

International Fund for Agricultural Development (IFAD). 2002c. *Valuing Diversity in Sustainable Development*. Rome: IFAD. Available online at: https://www.ifad.org/documents/10180/6370bd60-03d4-4cbf-afbf-12f9b4f75186

International Fund for Agricultural Development (IFAD). 2007. *Statistics and Key Facts about Indigenous Peoples*. Rome: IFAD. Available online at: http://www.ruralpoverty portal.org/web/guest/topic/statistics/tags/Indigenous%20peoples

International Fund for Agricultural Development (IFAD). 2010. Engagement with Indigenous Peoples. Rome: IFAD.

International Labour Organization (ILO). 1957. *International Labour Organization Convention (no. 107) concerning the Protection and Integration of Indigenous and Other Tribal and Semi-Tribal Populations in Independent Countries*. New York: United Nations Treaty Series.

International Labour Organization (ILO). 1989. *Indigenous and Tribal Peoples Convention*. C169, 27 June 1989, C169. Available online at: http://www.refworld.org/docid/3ddb6d514.html

International Symposium on the Social Determinants of Indigenous Health. 2007. *Social Determinants and Indigenous Health: The International Experience and Its Policy Implications*. Adelaide, Report for the Commission on Social Determinants of Health.

Inuit Tapiriit Kanatami. 2009. *Determinants of Inuit Health in Canada: A Discussion Paper*. Ottawa: Inuit Tapiriit Kanatami.

Inuit Women's Association. 1993. *A Response to the Articles of the Nunavut Proposal*. Copy Faxed: 10–27–93. Toronto: Inuit Women's Association.

Ioanid, R. 2000. *The Holocaust in Romania: The Destruction of Jews and Gypsies under the Antonescu Regime, 1940–1944*. Chicago, IL: Ivan R. D. Publisher Inc.

IPS. 1999. *Indigenous Struggle Continues in Latin America*. October 27. Italy:IPS.

Isaac, T. 1994. The concept of the crown and Aboriginal self-government. *Canadian Journal of Native Studies* 14(2): 221.

IUCN. 1997. *Indigenous Peoples and Sustainability: Cases and Actions, Inter-Commission Task Force on Indigenous Peoples*. Utrecht: International Books.

IWGIA. 2012. Indigenous World, 2012. Copenhagen: IWGIA.

IWGIA, 2013. Indigenous World, 2013. Copenhagen: IWGIA.

IWGIA, 2014. Indigenous World, 2014. Copenhagen: IWGIA.

Jack, S., Dobbins, M., Furgal, C., Greenwood, M., and Brooks, S. 2010. *Aboriginal Environmental Health Issues Researchers' and Decision-makers' Perceptions of Knowledge Transfer and Exchange Processes*. Prince George, British Columbia: National Collaborating Centre for Aboriginal Health, pp. 1–36.

Jacobs, M.A., and Saus, M. 2012. Child welfare services for Indigenous populations: A comparison of child welfare histories, policies, practices and laws for American Indians and Norwegian Sámis. *Child Care in Practice* 18(3): 271–290.

Janke, T. n.d. *Biodiversity, Patents and Indigenous Peoples*. Available online at: http://www.wacc.org.uk/de/content/pdf/1245 [Accessed on 12 March 2007].

Janz, T., Seto, J., and Turner, A. 2009. *Aboriginal Peoples Survey, 2006: An Overview of the Health of the Métis Population.* [Cat. No. 89-637-X-No. 004]. Ottawa, Ontario: Statistics Canada.

Jayanthi, V., Probert, C.S., Pinder, D., Wicks, A.C., and Mayberry, J.F. February 1992. Epidemiology of Crohn's disease in Indian migrants and the Indigenous population in Leicestershire. *Quarterly Journal of Medicine,* New Series 82(298): 125–138.

Jull, P. 1988. Building Nunavut: A story of Inuit self-government. *The Northern Review* 1(Summer): 59–72 (Canada).

Junghee, L., Donlan, W., Cardoso, E.E.O., and Paz, J.J. 2013. Cultural and social determinants of health among Indigenous Mexican migrants in the United States. *Social Work in Public Health* 28(6): 607–618.

Juutilainen, S.A., Miller, R., Heikkilä, L., and Rautio, A. 2014. Structural racism and Indigenous health: What Indigenous perspectives of residential school and boarding school tell us? A case study of Canada and Finland. *The International Indigenous Policy Journal* 5(3): 1–18.

Kalaydjieva, L., Morar, B., Chaix, R., and Tang, H. 2005. A newly discovered founder population: The Roma/Gypsies. *Bioessays* 27(10): 1084–1094.

Kaseje, D.A.N.C.O., Juma, P., and Oindo, M. 2005. Public health in Africa: What is new—The context, the gains, the losses, the renewed public health, and the way forward. *Kidney International* 68(Sept 98): S49–S59.

Keal, P. 2007. Indigenous self-determination and the legitimacy of sovereign states. *International Politics* 44: 287–305.

Kearney, M. 1995. The local and the global: The anthropology of globalization and transnationalism. *Annual Review of Anthropology* 24: 547–565.

Kelm, M. 1998. *Colonizing Bodies: Aboriginal Health and Healing in British Columbia, 1900–1950.* Vancouver: UBC Press.

Kirmayer, L.J., Brass, G.M., and Tait, C.L. 2000. The mental health of Aboriginal peoples: Transformations of identity and community. *Canadian Journal of Psychiatry* 45: 607–616.

Kishk Anaquot Health Research (KAHR). March 2008. *Structural Issues Affecting the World's Indigenous Peoples.* [Unpublished Report]. Ottawa, Canada: Canadian Coalition For Global Health Research.

Klein, H. 1982. Historia general de Bolivia. La Paz: Editorial Juventud.

Krieger, N. 2008. Proximal, distal, and the politics of causation: What's level got to do with it? *American Journal of Public Health* 98(2): 221–230.

Kuhnlein, H.V., and Receveur, O. 1996. Dietary change and traditional food systems of Indigenous peoples. *Annual Review in Nutrition* 16: 417–442.

Kunitz, J.S. 2000. Public health then and now: Globalization, states, and the health of Indigenous peoples. *American Journal of Public Health* 90: 1531–1539.

Kuokkanen, R. 17 June 2006. Sami Women, Autonomy and Decolonization in the Age of Globalization. *Keynote Speech at Rethinking Nordic Colonialism. A Postcolonial Exhibition Project in Five Acts. Act 4: Beyond Subject and State? Indigenous Interests in the Age of Globalization.* Rovaniemi: Arctic Center, University of Lapland. Available on: http://s3.amazonaws.com/academia.edu.documents/44482063/Kuokkanen.pdf?AWSAccessKeyId=AKIAJ56TQJRTWSMTNPEA&Expires=1474250398&Signature=pwfEEdXh5ny7appopnKRCwz%2B1j0%3D&response-content-disposition=inline%3B%20filename%3DSami_Women_Autonomy_and_Decolonization_i.pdf [Accessed on 16 January 2014].

Kukokkanen, R. 2008a. Globalization as racialized, sexualized violence. *International Feminist Journal of Politics* 10: 216–233, doi: 10.1080/14616740801957554.

Lang, T. 2001. Public health and colonialism: A new or old problem? *Journal of Epidemiology and Community Health* 55: 162–163. doi:10.1136/jech.55.3.162

LaRocque, E. 1993. Violence in Aboriginal Communities. In *The Path to Healing: Report of the National Round Table on Aboriginal Health and Social Issues*. A Paper prepared for the Royal Commission on Aboriginal Peoples. Vancouver, British Columbia: Minister of Supply and Services Canada, pp. 72–89.

Larsen, P.B. 2003. *Indigenous and Tribal Children: Assessing Child Labour and Education Challenges*. Geneva: International Labour Organization.

Lasimbang, J. 2008. Indigenous Peoples and Local Economic Development. Newsletter, Issue No. 5: 42–45. Chiangmai: *Asia Indigenous Peoples Pact* (AIPP).

Lavallee, C., and Bourgault, C. 2000. The health of Cree, Inuit and Southern Quebec women: Similarities and differences. *Canadian Journal of Public Health* 91: 212–216.

Lavoie, J., O'Neil, J., Reading, J., and Allard, Y. 1999. Community healing and Aboriginal self-government. In John H. Hylton (ed.), *Aboriginal Self-Government in Canada: Current Trends and Issues*, 2nd edn. Saskatoon: Purich Publishing, p. 130–147.

Lea, T. 2008. *Bureaucrats & Bleeding Hearts: Indigenous Health in the Northern Territory*. Sydney: UNSW Press.

Lee, J., Donlan, W., Cardoso, E.E.O., and Paz, J.J. 2013. Cultural and social determinants of health among Indigenous Mexican migrants in the United States. *Social Work in Public Health* 28(6): 607–618.

Lee, L., and Chen, P. 2014. Empowering Indigenous youth: Perspectives from a National Service Learning Program in Taiwan. *The International Indigenous Policy Journal* 5(3): 1–21.

Lehman, T.J.A. 2003. *Indigenous Peoples' Health: Why Are They Behind Everyone, Everywhere?* New York: Division of Pediatric Rheumatology, Hospital for Special Surgery, Weill Medical College of Cornell University.

Lewy, G. 2000. *The Nazi Persecution of the Gypsies*. New York, NY: Oxford University Press.

Lile, H.K. 2006. A new era for Indigenous peoples. *Gáldu Čála—Journal of Indigenous Peoples Rights* 2:10–12.

Linares, F.N. 2008. Los pueblos indígenas de México. México Comisión Nacional para el Desarrollo de los Pueblos Indígenas. Available on at: http://www.cdi.gob.mx/index.php?option=com_docman&itemid=24. [Retrieved 3 August 2009].

Linda, S. 2001. *Social and Economic Determinants of Health*. The Report of HIA on the Greater London Authority Draft Economic Development Strategy. London: HIA (Health Impact Assessment.

Ling, Y.V., and Raphael, D. 2004. Identifying and addressing the social determinants of the incidence and successful management of type 2 diabetes mellitus in Canada. *Canadian Journal of Public Health* 95(5): 366–368.

Little, L.M., and Prince, M.J. 1993. *Community Control of Health and Social Services in Northern and Aboriginal Communities: A Literature Review and Analysis of Canadian Experiences: Technical Report and Case Studies*. Northwest Territories: Legislative Assembly.

Lucas, K. 22 July 2005. Sick of globalization. *The Inter Press Service.*

Lucero, J.A. 2001. Crisis and contention in Ecuador. *Journal of Democracy* 12(2): 59–73.

Macaulay, A.C. 2009. Improving Aboriginal health: How can health care professionals contribute? Canadian Family Physician. Apr; 55(4): 334–336.

MacDonald, K.A. 2000. *First Nations Child and Family Services: Whither Self-Governance?* L.L.M. thesis, University of British Columbia.

Mackay, F. 2002. Universal rights or a universe unto itself? Indigenous peoples' human rights and the World Bank's draft operational policy on Indigenous peoples. *American University International Law Review* 528(17): 527.

MacKay, F. 28 June 2004. Indigenous peoples' right to free, prior and informed consent and the World Bank's extractive. *Industries Review* IV(2): 43–65.

Macklem, P. 1995. Normative dimensions of the right of Aboriginal self-government. Ottawa: Minister of Supply and Services.

MacMillan, H.L., Jamieson, E., Walsh, C.A., Wong, M.Y.Y., Faries, E.J., McCue, H., et al. 2008. First Nations women's mental health: Results from an Ontario survey. *Archives of Women's Mental Health* 11: 109–15.

MacMillan, H.L., Walsh, C.A., Jamieson, E., Wong, M.Y.Y., Faries, E.J., McCue, H., A.B. MacMillan, D.R. Offord. 2003. The health of Ontario First Nations people: Results from the Ontario First Nations Regional Health Survey. *Canadian Journal of Public Health* 94(3): 168–72.

Mander, J., and Tauli-Corpuz, V. (Eds.) 2006. *Paradigm wars: Indigenous Peoples' Resistance to Globalization.* San Francisco: Sierra Club Books.

Manning, R., and Puruntatameri, B. 2005. *Effective Community Control: The Way Forward for Improving Indigenous Health.* Paper presented to the 8th National Rural Health Conference, Alice Springs, Northern Territory, March 10–13.

Martínez-Cobo, J. 1986/87. Study of the Problem of Discrimination against Indigenous Populations. Prepared by Special Rapporteur to the Subcommission on Prevention of Discrimination and Protection of Minorities. UN DOC E/CN.4/ Sub.2/1986/7; see http://www.un.org/esa/socdev/unpfii.

Martínez Cobo, J. 1986/7. *Study of the Problem of Discrimination against Indigenous Populations.* UN Doc. E/CN.4/Sub.2/1986/7 and Add. 1–4. Available online at: http://www.un.org/esa/socdev/unpfii/en/second.html

Martinez, J.M.A. 2012. Indigenous peoples' struggles for autonomy: The case of the U'wa people. *Paterson Review of International Affairs* 12: 109–122.

Mattiace, S. 2000. *Multiculturalism in (Post) Modern Mexico: Making Subjects or Subject Making? A View from Las Margaritas, Chiapas.* Paper delivered at the Congress of the Latin American Studies Association.

McDonald, C. 2013. Poverty in Australia and the social work response. *Asia Pacific Journal of Social Work and Development* 23(1): 3–11.

McDonnell, R., and Depew, R. 1999. Aboriginal self-government and self-determination in Canada: A critical commentary. In John H. Hylton (ed.), *Aboriginal Self-Government in Canada: Current Trends and Issues*, 2nd edn. Saskatoon: Purich Publishing, p. 352–372.

McIntyre, L. 2004. Food insecurity. In D. Raphael (ed.), *Social Determinants of Health: Canadian Perspectives.* Toronto: Canadian Scholars' Press Inc., pp. 188–204.

McNeil, K. 2001–2002. Self-government and the inalienability of Aboriginal title. *McGill Law Journal* 47: 473.

Micha, J.M. 2012. Strategies on Implementing Self-Government, March 29. Ottawa: Action Canada.

Ministère de la Sécurité du revenu du Québec (MSRQ). 1995. *Profil des personnes autochtones aptes au travail, à l'aide de dernier recours.* Québec: Direction générale des politiques et des programmes, Direction de la recherche, de l'évaluation et de la statistique.

Minority Rights Group International. June 2008. *World Directory of Minorities and Indigenous Peoples – Ethiopia: Overview.* Available online at: http://www.refworld.org/docid/4954ce295.html [Accessed on 09 April 2011].

Mohsin, A. 2000. State hegemony. In P. Gain (ed.), *The Chittagong Hill Tracts: Life and Nature at Risk.* Dhaka: Society for Environmental and Human Development (SEHD), pp. 59–77.

Mokuau, N. 2011. Culturally based solutions to preserve the health of native Hawaiians. *Journal of Ethnic and Cultural Diversity in Social Work* 20(2): 98–113.

Moran, M.F. 2004. The practice of participatory planning at Mapoon Aboriginal settlement: Towards community control, ownership and autonomy. *Australian Geographical Studies* 43(3): 339–355.

Moreton-Robinson, A. 2006. Towards a new research agenda? Foucault, whiteness and Indigenous sovereignty. *Journal of Sociology* 42(4): 383–395.

Morrissey, M. 2002. Poverty and Indigenous health: Notes for workshop on social determinants of health. Mezies School of Health Research, 3 June. Darwin: Menzies School of Health Research.

Morse, B. 1999. The inherent right of Aboriginal governance. In John H. Hylton (ed.), *Aboriginal Self-Government in Canada: Current Trends and Issues*, 2nd edn. Saskatoon: Purich Publishing, pp. 16–44.

Moss, W. 1995. Inuit perspectives on treaty rights and governance. In Patrick M, et al (Eds) *Aboriginal Self-Government: Legal and Constitutional Issues*. Ottawa: Royal Commission on Aboriginal Peoples, Minister of Supply and Services Canada.

Mussell, W.J., Nicholls, W.M., and Adler, M.T. 1993. *Making Meaning of Mental Health: Challenges in First Nations*, 2nd edn. Chilliwack, British Columbia: Sal'I'shan Institute.

Naim, M. 2003. *An Indigenous World: How Native Peoples Can Turn Globalization to their Advantage.* Available online at: https://www.globalpolicy.org/globaliz/politics/2003/12moisesnaim.htm

Nash, June. 2003. Indigenous development alternatives. *Urban Anthropology* 32(1): 57–72.

National Collaborating Centre for Aboriginal Health. 2007a. Exploring Evidence in Aboriginal Health. In *Proceedings from the Indigenous Knowledge Dialogue Circle, Vancouver BC*. Prince George, British Columbia: National Collaborating Centre for Aboriginal Health, pp. 1–6.

National Collaborating Centre for Aboriginal Health. 2007b. *Landscapes of Indigenous Health: An Environmental Scan by the NCCAH*. Prince George, British Columbia: National Collaborating Centre for Aboriginal Health.

National Collaborating Centre for Aboriginal Health. 2009. *Culture and Language as Social Determinants of First Nations, Inuit and Métis Health*. Prince George, British Columbia: National Collaborating Centre for Aboriginal Health.

Native Women's Association of Canada. 2002. *Aboriginal Women and Health Care in Canada*. Ottawa, Ontario: Native Women's Association of Canada.

Native Women's Association of Canada. 2004. *Background Document on Aboriginal Women's Health for the Health Sectoral Session, Following up to the Canada-Aboriginal Peoples Roundtable*. Ottawa, Ontario: Native Women's Association of Canada.

Native Women's Association of Canada (NWAC). 4 June 2007. *Social Determinants of Health and Canada's Aboriginal Women Submission by the Native Women's Association of Canada to the World Health Organization's Commission on the Social Determinants of Health*. Ottawa: NWAC.

Netherlands Centre for Indigenous Peoples (NCIP). 2010. *Definition of Indigenous Peoples. Updates*. Netherlands. Available online at: http://Indigenouspeoples.nl/Indigenous-peoples/definition-Indigenous

Newhouse, D.R., and Belanger, Y.D. 2001. *Aboriginal Self-Government in Canada, A Review of Literature since 1960*. [Unpublished]. Native Studies, Trent University.

Niezen, R. 2003. *The Origins of Indigenism: Human Rights and the Politics of Identity.* Berkeley, CA: University of California Press.

North, D. 1990. *Institutions, Institutional Change and Economic Performance.* Cambridge: Cambridge University Press.OHCHR. 2014. Report of the Special Rapporteur on the rights of indigenous peoples, James Anaya. Available on http://www.ohchr.org/Documents/Issues/IPeoples/SR/A.HRC.27.52.Add.2-MissionCanada_AUV.pdf [Accessed on 3 June 2016].

OHCHR. 2015. Report of the Special Rapporteur on the rights of Indigenous peoples, Victoria Tauli-Corpuz, regarding the situation of Indigenous peoples in Paraguay. Geneva: OHCHR. available on www.ohchr.org/EN/HRBodies/HRC/. . ./A_HRC_30_41_Add_1_ENG-.docx

Olivera, M. 2012. The Gypsies as Indigenous groups: The Gabori Roma case in Romania. *Romani Studies* 22(1): 19–33.

Ompad, D.C., Galea, S., Caiaffa, W. T., and Vlahov, D. 2007. Social determinants of the health of urban populations: Methodologic considerations. *Journal of Urban Health* 84(1): 42–53.

Osman, S. 2000. Globalization and democratization: The response of the Indigenous people of Sarawak. *Third World Quarterly* 21(6): 977–988.

Oviawe, J.O. 2013. *Appropriating Colonialism: Complexity And Chaos In The Making Of A Nigeria-Centric Educational System.* Unpublished PhD thesis. Washington State University, Washington.

Oxfam. 2006. *Programme Overview.* Dhaka: Oxfam in Bangladesh.

Pan American Health Organization, and the World Health Organization. 2006. *Health of the Indigenous Population in the Americas.* Washington: PAHO.

Patwardhan, A. 2007. *Dams and Tribal People in India.* Contributing Paper prepared for Thematic Review 1.2: Dams, Indigenous People and Vulnerable Ethnic Minorities. World Commission on Dams.

Peeler, J. 2000. *Citizenship and Difference: Indigenous Politics in Guatemala and the Central Andes.* Paper delivered at the Congress of the Latin American Studies Association.

Peeling, A.C., and Chartrand, Paul L.A.H. 2004. Sovereignty, liberty, and the legal order of the 'freemen': Towards a constitutional theory of Métis self-government. *Saskatchewan Law Review* 67: 339.

Penikett, T. 2012a. A 'Literacy Test' for Indigenous government? *Northern Public Affairs*, 1.1: 32–37.

Penikett, T. 2012b. *Six Definitions of Aboriginal Self-Government and the Unique Haida Model.* Paper prepared for the Action Canada Northern Conference, Haida Gwaii, September 2012.

Penner, K. 1983. *Indian Self-Government.* Ottawa: House of Commons.

Peters, E.J. 1999. Geographies of Aboriginal self-government. In John H. Hylton (ed.), *Aboriginal Self-Government in Canada: Current Trends and Issues*, 2nd edn. Saskatoon: Purich Publishing, pp. 411–431.

Pettifer, C. 1993. Métis Child and Family Services. In *The Path to Healing: Report of the National Round Table on Aboriginal Health and Social Issues.* A Paper prepared for the Royal Commission on Aboriginal Peoples. Vancouver, British Columbia: Canadian Cataloguing in Publication Data, pp. 224–226.

Porter, D. 1999. *Health, Civilization and the State: A History of Public Health From Ancient to Modern Times.* London: Routledge.

Postero, N. 2000. *Bolivia's Indígena Citizen: Multiculturalism in a Neoliberal Age.* Paper delivered at the Congress of the Latin American Studies Association.

Postl, B., Cook, C., and, Moffatt, M.E. 2010. Aboriginal child health and the social determinants: why are these children so disadvantaged? *Healthcare Quarterly* 14(1): 42–51.

Psachaopoulos, G., and Patrinos, H.A. 1994. *Indigenous People and Poverty in Latin America: An Empirical Analysis.* Washington, DC: The World Bank.

Pulver, L.R., Jackson, E.H., and Waldon, J. 2015. An overview of the existing knowledge on the social determinants of Indigenous health and well being in Australia and New Zealand. DOI: 10.13140/RG.2.1.4415.2803 (also available here http://www.pha.org.nz/documents/gnoverview.pdf

Putt, J. January 2013. *Conducting Research with Indigenous People and Communities.* Brief 15. New South Wales, Australia: The Indigenous Justice Clearinghouse.

Radcliffe, S., Laurie, N. and, Andolina, R. 28 February 2002. *Indigenous People and Political Transnationalism: Globalization from Below Meets Globalization from Above.* Paper presented to the Transnational Communities Programme Seminar, held at the School of Geography, University of Oxford.

Rady, M. 1992. *Romania in Turmoil.* New York, NY: IB Tauris and Co. Ltd.

The Rain Forest Action Network. 2001, January. In Defense of Sacred Lands : The Uwa People's Struggle Against Big Oil. Available online at: http://www.wellnessgoods.com/defensesacredlands.asp [Accessed on 23 September 2015].

Ramasubramanian, R. 2005. *Elusive Peace in the Chittagong Hill Tracts: A Backgrounder.* [Paper No. 1540]. Delhi: South Asia Analysis Group.

Ranger, T. October 2003. Christianity and Indigenous peoples: A personal overview. *The Journal of Religious History* 27(3): 255–271.

Raphael, D. 2001. *Inequality is Bad for Our Hearts: Why Low Income and Social Exclusion Are Major Causes of Heart Disease in Canada.* Toronto: North York Heart Network.

Raphael, D. 2002. *Social Determinants of Health: Why Is There Such a Gap between Our Knowledge and Its Implementation?* Available online at: http://www.medanthro.net/academic/topical/ryerson.ppt#1 [Accessed on 6 December 2010].

Raphael, D. 2004. Introduction to the social determinants of health. In D. Raphael (ed.), *Social Determinants of Health: Canadian Perspectives.* Toronto: Canadian Scholars' Press Inc., pp. 2–18.

Reading, C.L., and Wien, F. 2009. *Health Inequalities and Social Determinants of Aboriginal Peoples' Health.* Prince George, British Columbia: National Collaborating Centre for Aboriginal Health, University of Northern British Columbia.

Reading, J., and Nowgesic, E. 2002. Improving the health of future generations: The Canadian Institutes of Health Research Institute of Aboriginal Peoples' health. *American Journal of Public Health* 92(9): 1396–1400.

Reading, J., Ritchie, A.J., Victor, J.C., and Wilson, E. 2005. Implementing empowering health promotion programmes for Aboriginal youth in two distinct communities in British Columbia, Canada. *Promotion & Education* 12: 62–65.

Reinsborough, P. 2002. Victory for the U'wa. *Earth First! Journal.* Available online at: http://www.earthfirstjournal.org/article.php?id=130.

Richmond, C.A.M, and Ross, N.A. 2008. Social support, material circumstance and health behavior: Influences on health in First Nation and Inuit communities of Canada. *Social Science and Medicine* 67: 1423–1433.

Richmond, C.A.M., and Ross, N.A. 2009. The determinants of First Nation and Inuit health: A critical population health approach. *Health & Place* 15: 403–411.

Richmond, C.A.M., Ross, N.A., and Egeland, G.M. 2007. Social support and thriving health: A new approach to understanding the health of Indigenous Canadians. *American Journal of Public Health* 97: 1827–1833.

Riecken, T., Scott, T., and Tanaka, M.T. 2006. Community and culture as foundations for resilience: Participatory health research with First Nations student filmmakers. *Journal of Aboriginal Health* 3: 7–14.

Riley, M. 2000. *Nutritional Health of Indigenous Peoples: Whose Responsibility? Asia Pacific Journal of Clinical Nutrition* 9(3): 155–156

Rist, G. 1997. *The History of Development: From Western Origins to Global Faith.* London: Zed Books.

Rivers, D.S. 2005. *Zapotec Use of E-Commerce: The Portrait of Teotitlan Del Valle, Mexico.* Unpublished PhD dissertation. Michigan State University, East Lansing, MI. Publication No. AAT 3216168. Available at: ABI/INFORM Global database [Accessed 16 January 2014].

Robbins, J.A., and Dewar, J. 2011. Traditional Indigenous approaches to healing and the modern welfare of traditional knowledge, spirituality and lands: A critical reflection on practices and policies taken from the Canadian Indigenous example. *The International Indigenous Policy Journal* 2(4): 2–17.

Rodríguez-Garavito, C.A., and Arenas, L.C. 2005. Indigenous rights, transnational activism, and legal mobilization: The struggle of the U'wa people in Colombia. In Boaventura de Sousa Santos and César A. Rodríguez-Garavito (eds.), *Law and Globalization from Below: Towards a Cosmopolitan Legality.* New York: Cambridge University Press, pp. 241–266.

Rodríguez-Garavito, C. 2010. Ethnicity.gov: Global governance, Indigenous peoples, and the right to prior consultation in social minefields. *Indiana Journal of Global Legal Studies* 18(1):1–44.

Ron, B. 2001. Australian Indigenous mental health. *Australian and New Zealand Journal of Mental Health Nursing* 10: 33–41.

Roy, R.C.K. 2000. *Land Rights of the Indigenous Peoples of the Chittagong Hill Tracts* Copenhagen: IWGIA.

Roy, R.D. 2003. The discordant accord: Challenges towards the implementation of the Chittagong Hill Tracts Accord of 1997. *Journal of Social Studies* 100: 6 (University of Dhaka).

Roy, R.D. 2010. *Country Technical Notes on Indigenous Peoples' Issues: Bangladesh.* Italy: IFAD.

Royal Commission on Aboriginal Peoples (RCAP). 1993. *Sharing the Harvest, the Road to Self-Reliance.* Report of the National Round Table on Aboriginal Development and Resources. Ottawa: Supply and Services Canada.

Royal Commission on Aboriginal Peoples (RCAP). 1996. *Report of the Royal Commission on Aboriginal Peoples: Volume 2. Restructuring the Relationship.* Ottawa: RCAP.

Russell, V.L., and de Leeuw, S. March 2012. Aboriginal women's lived experiences of health services in Northern British Columbia and the potential of creative arts to raise awareness about HPV, cervical cancer, and screening. *Journal of Aboriginal Health* 8(1): 18–27.

SACOSS (South Australian Council of Social Sciences). 2007. Blueprint for the eradication of poverty in South Australia. Unley: SACOSS.

Sadik, N. 23 July 2013. Israel's Bedouin population faces mass eviction. *New Internationalist.* Available online at: http://newint.org/features/web-exclusive/2013/07/23/bedouins-face-mass-eviction/

Sakuda, F.N.O. Fall 2004. The hardships and successes of being Indigenous in Africa. *CSQ* 28(3): 1–5 (The International Decade of the World's Indigenous People).

Sanborne, M. 1996. *Nations in Transition: Romania.* New York, NY: Facts on File Inc.

Santos, R. 24 July 2010. The Maasai tribe goes mobile. *2010 Global Marketing*. Available online at: http://2010globalmarketing.wordpress.com/2010/07/24/695/.

Sara, J.M. 2006. *Indigenous Governance of Self-Determination. The Saami Model and the Saami Parliament in Norway*. Symposium on 'The Right to Self-Determination in International Law' Organised by Unrepresented Nations and Peoples Organization (UNPO), Khmers Kampuchea-Krom Federation (KKF), Hawai'i Institute for Human Rights (HIHR), The Hague, Netherlands, 29 September–1 October.

Scarpa, F. May 2013. *The EU, the Arctic and Arctic Indigenous Peoples*. Unpublished Master's thesis. University of Akureyri, Faculty of Law and Social Sciences, Department of Law, Iceland.

Scholte, J.A. 2000. *Globalization: A Critical Introduction*. New York: St. Martin's Press.

Schroeder, K. 2007. Economic globalization and Bolivia's regional divide. *Journal of Latin American Geography* 6(2): 99–120.

Scott, K.A. 1993. Funding Policy for Indigenous Human Services. In *The Path to Healing: Report to the National Round Table on Aboriginal Health and Social Issues*. Royal Commission on Aboriginal Peoples, pp. 90–107.

Shah, A. 9 December 2006. Rights of Indigenous people. *Global Issues*. Available at: http://www.globalissues.org/article/693/rights-of-Indigenous-people [Accessed on 22 May 2015].

Shah, B.R., Gunraj, N., and Hux, J.E. May 2003. Markers of access to and quality of primary care for Aboriginal people in Ontario, Canada. *American Journal of Public Health* 93(5): 798–802.

Shastri, V. 2007. *Migration of Aryans from India*. Varanasi: Yogic Voice Consciousness Institute.

Shanker, J., Ip, E., Khamela, E., Couture, J., Tan, S., Zulla, R.T., and Lam, G. 2013. Education as a social determinant of health: Issues facing Indigenous and visible minority students in postsecondary education in western Canada. *International Journal of Environment Research in Public Health* 10(Sept 9): 3908–3929.

Shepherd, C.C.J., Li, J., and Zubrick, S.R. 2012. Social gradients in the health of Indigenous Australians. *American Journal of Public Health* 102(1): 107–117.

Sheridan, L. 2001. Social and economic determinants of health. The report of HIA on the Greater London Authority draft economic development strategy. London: HIA (Health Impact Assessment.

Shewell, H. 1995. The First Nations of Canada: Social welfare and the quest for self-government. In J. Dixon and R.P. Scheurell (eds.), *Social Welfare and Indigenous Peoples*. London and New York: Routledge, pp. 1–53.

Sibbald, B. 2002. Off-reserve Aboriginal people face daunting health problems: *Canadian Medical Association Journal* 167: 912.

Sinclair, R., Smith, R., and Stevenson, N. 2006. *Miyo-Mahcihowin: A Report on Indigenous Health in Saskatchewan*. Regina, Saskatchewan: Indigenous Peoples Health Research Centre.

Singh, R. 1996. The Chittagong Hill Tracts in Bangladesh. In: C. Nicholas and R. Singh (eds.), *Indigenous Peoples of Asia: Many Peoples, One Struggle*. Bangkok: Asia Indigenous Peoples Pact.

Sinha, V., and Kozlowski, A. 2013. The structure of Aboriginal child welfare in Canada. *The International Indigenous Policy Journal* 4(2): 1–21.

Slowey, G.A. 2005. Globalization and Development in the Fourth World: Indigenous Experiences in Canada and New Zealand Compared. Paper Prepared for the 4th International Critical Management Studies Conference, 4-6 July 2005. University of Cambridge, Cambridge, UK.

Smith, J., and Kroondyk, J. March 2009. *We'll Trade You Cheap Labor for Cheap Labor-ers: How Trade Policies Impact Immigration.* Presented at the 10th Conference on Americas, Grand Rapids, Michigan.

Smith, L.T. 2008. *Decolonizing Methodologies: Research and Indigenous Peoples.* London and New York: Zed Books Ltd. and Dunedin: University of Otago Press.

Smylie, J. 2009–2010. *Achieving Strength through Numbers: First Nations, Inuit, and Metis Health Information.* Prince George, British Columbia: National Collaborating Centre for Aboriginal Health, pp. 1–4.

Snipp, M.C. 1989. *American Indians: The First of This Land.* New York: Russell Sage Foundation.

Stanton, K. 2011. Canada's Truth and Reconciliation Commission: Settling the past?. *The International Indigenous Policy Journal* 2(3): 1–20.

Statistics Canada. 1993. *Schooling, Work and Related Activities, Income, Expenses and Mobility.* Ottawa: Minister of Industry, Science and Technology.

Statistics Canada. May 1998. *An Overview of Data on Aboriginal Peoples.* Canadian Centre for Justice Statistics Bulletin. Ottawa: Statistcs Canada.

Statistics Canada. 9 November 1999. General social survey: Time use. *The Daily.* Available online at: http://www.statcan.ca/Daily/English/991109/td991109.htm

Statistics Canada. January 2000a. *Police-Reported Aboriginal Crime in Saskatchewan.* Canadian Centre for Justice Statistics. [Cat. No. 85F0031XIE].

Statistics Canada. 2000b. *How Healthy are Canadians? A Summary.* Ottawa: Statistics Canada, Health Statistics Division. Available online at: http://www.statcan.ca/english/ads/82–003-XIB/summary11–3.pdf

Statistics Canada. 2001a. *A Portrait of Aboriginal Children Living in Non-reserve Areas: Results from the 2001 Aboriginal Peoples Survey.* [Cat. No. 89-597-XIE]. Canada.

Statistics Canada. 2001b. *Aboriginal Peoples of Canada 2001 Census.* Ottawa: Statistics Canada.

Statistics Canada. 2005. Projections of the Aboriginal Populations, Canada, Provinces and Territories. Catalogue no. 91-547-XIE, Ottawa: Statistics Canada.

Statistics Canada. 2008. *Social and Aboriginal Statistics Division. Aboriginal Peoples Survey, 2006: Inuit Health and Social Conditions.* Ottawa, Ontario.

Statistics Canada. 2009. *Aboriginal Peoples Survey, 2006. An Overview of the Health of the Métis Population.* Available online at: http://www.statcan.gc.ca/pub/89-637-x/89-637-x2009004-eng.htm [Accessed on 1 November 2011].

Statistics Canada. 2014. Victimization of Aboriginal people in Canada, 2014. Ottawa: Statistics Canada.

Stavenhagen, R. 1996. Indigenous rights: Some conceptual problems. In E. Jelin and E. Hershberg (eds.), *Constructing Democracy: Human Rights, Citizenship, and Society in Latin America.* Boulder, CO: Westview Press, pp. 141–159.

Stavenhagen, R. 2003. *Indigenous Peoples and their Access to Human Rights.* Paper Presented at the International Council on Human Rights Policy. Sixth Annual Assembly Access to Human Rights: Improving Access for Groups at High Risk, Guadalajara, January 17–18.

Stavenhagen, R. 2005. *Indigenous Peoples: Land, Territory, Autonomy, and Self-Determination.* UN Special Rapporteur on the Situation of the Human Rights and Fundamental Freedoms of Indigenous Peoples.

Stewart, J., and Allan, J. 2013. Building relationships with Aboriginal people: A cultural mapping toolbox. *Australian Social Work* 66(1): 118–129.

Stewart, M. 1997. *The Time of the Gypsies.* Boulder, CO: Westview Press.

Stout, M.D., Kipling, G.D., Stout, R., and Centres of Excellence for Women's Health Research Synthesis Group. 2001. *Aboriginal Women's Health Research Synthesis Project: Final Report*. Vancouver, British Columbia: British Columbia Centre of Excellence for Women's Health, BC Women's Hospital and Health Centre. Available online at: http://www.cewh-cesf.ca/PDF/cross_cex/synthesisEN.pdf

Stout, R., and Harp, R. 2009. *Aboriginal Maternal and Infant Health in Canada: Review of On-Reserve Programming*. Available online at: http://www.pwhce.ca/pdf/Aborig Maternal_programmes.pdf [Accessed on 8 November 2011].

Strom, Y. 1993. *Uncertain Roads: Searching for the Gypsies*. New York, NY: Four Winds Press, MacMillan Publishing Co.

Suagee, D.B., and Stearns, C.T. 1994. Indigenous self-government, environmental protection, and the consent of the governed: A tribal environmental review process. *Colorado Journal of International Environmental Law and Policy* 5(1): 59–104.

Tanner, A. 2001. The double bind of Aboriginal self-government. In Colin H. Scott (ed.), *Aboriginal Autonomy and Development in Northern Quebec and Labrador*. Vancouver: UBC Press, pp. 396–413.

Tashev, T., and Bechev, T. 2007. Bulgaria. In M. Nicoara (ed.), *Decade Watch: Roma Activists Assess the Progress of the Decade of Roma Inclusion 2005–2006*. Hungary: Createch Ltd., pp. 57–66.

Tauli-Corpuz, V. 2005. Indigenous peoples and the millennium development goals. *Indigenous Perspectives* VII(1): 3–28 (Tebtebba Foundation).

Tavanti, M. 2003, April 13. *Globalization Effects in Chiapas, Mexico*. The Midwest Worker. Available online at: http://www.jubilee4justice.org/Globalization_effects_in_Chiapas_Mexico.pdf [Accessed on 6 January 2014].

Taylor-Henley, S., and Hudson, P. 1992. Aboriginal self-government and social services: First Nations—provincial relationships. *Canadian Public Policy Analyse de Politiques* XVIII(1): 13–26.

Te Ata o Tu MacDonald, L., and Muldoon, P. 2006. Globalisation, neo-liberalism and the struggle for Indigenous citizenship. *Australian Journal of Political Science* 41(2): 209–23.

Tebtebba Foundation. 2004. *Forest Peoples Programs. Extracting Promises: Indigenous Peoples, Extractive Industries & the World Bank*. Baguio City: Tebtebba Foundation.

Time. 11 April 2016. *Suicide crisis in remote community puts spotlight on Aboriginal Canadians*. Available online at: http://time.com/4288086/canada-aboriginal-community-suicide-attawapiskat/

Timpson, J., Semple, D., and The Shibogama First Nations Council. 1997. Bringing home Payahtakenemowin (Peace of Mind): Creating self-government community services. *Native Social Work Journal* 1(1): 87–101.

Tompa, E., Polanyi, M., and Foley, J. 2004. Labour market flexibility and worker insecurity. In D. Raphael (ed.), *Social Determinants of Health: Canadian Perspectives*. Toronto: Canadian Scholars' Press Inc., pp. 88–98.

Townsend, P., Davidson, N., and Whitehead, M. (Eds.). 1992. *Inequalities in Health: The Black Report and the Health Divide*. London: Penguin Books.

Tse, S., Lloyd, C., Petchkovsky, L., and Manaia, W. 2005. Indigenous spirituality and mental health Exploration of Australian and New Zealand Indigenous people's spirituality and mental health. *Australian Occupational Therapy Journal* 52: 181–187.

Tully, J. 2000. Aboriginal peoples: Negotiating reconciliation. In J. Bickerton and A.G. Gagnon (eds.), *Canadian Politics*, 3rd edn. Peterborough: Broadview Press.

Ullah, AKM Ahsan and Labonte R. 2007. Globalization and the health of Indigenous peoples: From colonization to self-rule. Institute of Population Health. University of Ottawa. Canada. August. [Unpublished report]

Ullah, AKM Ahsan, and Routray, J.K. 2007. Rural poverty alleviation through NGO interventions in Bangladesh: How far is the achievement? *International Journal of Social Economics* 34(4): 237–248.

Ullah, AKM Ahsan. 2014. *Refugee Politics in the Middle East and the Africa: Human Rights, Safety and Identity.* London: Palgrave McMillan.

Ulloa, A. 2003. *The Ecological Native: Indigenous Peoples' Movements and Eco-Governmentality in Colombia.* Paper presented at the 2003 Meeting of the Latin American Studies Association, Dallas, Texas, March 27–29.

UN. 2007. *United Nations Declaration on the Rights of Indigenous Peoples.* 107th plenary meeting. New York: UN.

UN. 2008. *United Nations Declaration on the Rights of Indigenous Peoples.* Available online at: http://www.un.org/esa/socdev/unpfii/documents/DRIPS_en.pdf

UN. 2009. *Rethinking Poverty Report on the World Social Situation 2010.* New York: Department of Economic and Social Affairs, United Nations.

UN. 2010. *Urban Indigenous Peoples and Migration: A Review of Policies and Practices.* Available online at: http://www.unhabitat.org/pmss/listItemDetails.aspx?publication ID=2916.

UNDP. 2002. *Avoiding the Dependency Trap.* Bratislava, Slovak Republic: UNDP.

UNDP. 2006. At Risk: The Social Vulnerability of Roma, Refugees and Internally Displaced Persons in Serbia. June. Belgrade: UNDP.

UNDP. 2010. Indigenous Peoples in the Philippines. Fast Fact, February. The Philippines: UNDP.

UNDRIP, 2007. 61/295. United Nations Declaration on the Rights of Indigenous Peoples. Ney York: United Nations.

Ungerleider, C., and Burns, T. 2004. The state and quality of Canadian public education. In D. Raphael (ed.), *Social Determinants of Health: Canadian Perspectives.* Toronto: Canadian Scholars' Press Inc., pp. 156–169.

UNHCR. 2011. Mindanao's Indigenous people ask UNHCR's help to gain their rights. 10 October. Available online at:http://www.unhcr.org/news/latest/2011/10/4e92fc216/ mindanaos-indigenous-people-ask-unhcrs-help-gain-rights.html. [Accessed May 2016].

UNHRC. 2015. *UNHCR Statistical Online Population Database.* Available online at: www.unhcr.org/statistics/populationdatabase

United Nations. 2005. *Permanent Forum on Indigenous Issues.* Fourth Session. 8th Meeting (AM). 20/5/2005. HR/4842 United Nations.

United Nations. March 2006. *Indigenous Issues: Human Rights and Indigenous Issues.* Report of the Special Rapporteur on the Situation of Human Rights and Fundamental Freedoms of Indigenous People, Mission to New Zealand. GE.06–11836. Geneva.

United Nations Declaration on the Rights of Indigenous Peoples. *Strategic Comments* 12.8 (2007): 1–2. *United Nations Declaration on the Rights of Indigenous Peoples.* United Nations. Available online at: http://www.un.org/esa/socdev/unpfii/documents/ DRIPS_en.pdf

United Nations Department of Economics & Social Affairs. 2009. *State of the World's Indigenous Peoples.* New York: United Nations, pp. 4–7. Available online at: http:// www.un.org/esa/socdev/unpfii/documents/SOWIP_web.pdf

United Nations Department of Public Information. 2010. *State of the World's Indigenous People.* Available online at: http://www.un.org/esa/socdev/unpfii/documents/SOWIP_ Press_package.pdf

United Nations, Economic and Social Council (ECOSOC). 21 May 1971. *The Problem of Indigenous Populations*. Res. 1589(L) 7, U.N. Doc. E/5044.

United Nations Educational, Scientific, and Cultural Organization (UNESCO). 21 February 2012. *The Interactive Atlas of Endangered Languages*. Available online at: http://www.unesco.org/new/en/media-services/single-view/news/the_interactive_atlas_of_endangered_languages_updates/#.Usv2oWQW1xs

UNHR. 2013. *Indigenous Peoples and the United Nations Human Rights System*. Fact Sheet No. 9/Rev.2. Geneva: UNHR.

United Nations Permanent Forum on Indigenous Issues. n.d. *Indigenous Peoples, Indigenous Voices*. Available online at: www.un.org/esa/socdev/unpfii/documents/5session_factsheet1.pdf

United Nations Permanent Forum on Indigenous Issues. May 2006. *Indigenous Peoples, Indigenous Voices Factsheet: Indigenous Peoples and Identity*. Special Theme: The Millennium Development Goals and Indigenous Peoples: Re-defining the Millennium Development Goals. United Nations.

United Nations Permanent Forum on Indigenous Issues. 2007. *Indigenous Peoples – Lands, Territories and Natural Resources: Backgrounder*. United Nations.

United Nations Permanent Forum on Indigenous Issues. 2014. *Indigenous Peoples and the Millennium Development Goals*. Available online at: www.un.org/esa/socdev/unpfii/en/mdgs.html [Accessed on 12 July 2014].

United Nations Press Release. 2010. *State of the World's Indigenous Peoples*. Available online at: www.un.org/esa/socdev/unpfii/documents/SOWIP_Press_package.pdf

UNPFII. 2010. Permanent Forum on Indigenous Issues Report on the ninth session (19–30 April). Supplement No. 23. UNPFII: New York.

UNPFII Factsheet, 2010. Who are indigenous peoples? UNPFII: New York: UNPFII.

UNPFII. 2014. Indigenous Peoples and the Millennium Development Goals. Retrieved 12 July 2014, from www.un.org/esa/socdev/unpfii/en/mdgs.html

US Census. 2012. The American Indian and Alaska Native Population, 2010 Census Briefs, C2010BR-10. Washington: US Census Bureau.

Van Wagner, V., Epoo, B., Nastapoka, J., and Harney, E. 2007. Reclaiming birth, health, and community: Midwifery in the Inuit villages of Nunavik, Canada. *Journal of Midwifery & Women's Health* 52: 384–391.

Varennes, Fernand de. 2012. Language, Rights and Opportunities: The Role of Language in the Inclusion and Exclusion of Indigenous Peoples. Canada: Faculty of Law, Université de Moncton.

Venne, S.H. 1998. *Our Elders Understand Our Rights: Evolving International Law Regarding Indigenous Peoples*. Penticton, British Columbia: Theytus Books.

Veronica, A., Arnott, A., Ayre, M., Blohm, R., Grenfell, M., Purdon, A., Vemuri, R., and Wearne, G. 2005. *Negotiating Work: Indigenous Labour Market Report and Development Plan*. Canberra, Australia: Commonwealth Department of Transport and Regional Services.

Villarreal, M.A., and Fergusson, I.F. 2015. *The North American Free Trade Agreement (NAFTA)*. April 16. (CRS) Congressional Research Service. Report. R42965. Washington: CRS.

Wagner, R. 1998. *La conformación del Estado Guatemalteco*. Guatemala: Associate for Research on Social Studies.

Waldon, J. 2010. Tamariki Māori: A Māori view of children's rights. Working Paper. August. New Zealand: Action for Children and Youth Aotearoa.

Walker, J., and McDonald, D. August 1995. The over-representation of Indigenous people in custody in Australia. *Trends and Issues in Crime and Criminal Justice* 47: 2–6.

Walker, M., Fredericks, B., Mills, K., and Anderson, D. 2014. 'Yarning' as a method for community-based health research with Indigenous women: The Indigenous Women's Wellness Research Program. *Health Care for Women International* 35(10): 1216–1226.

Wall, D. 1998. *Aboriginal self-government in Canada: The Cases of Nunavut and the Alberta Métis Settlements*. Canada: Parliament Library.

Walter, M. 2007. Aboriginality, poverty and health—exploring the connections. In B. Carson, T. Dunbar, R.D. Chenall, and R. Baile (eds.), *Social Determinants of Indigenous Health*. Australia: Allen & Unwin, pp. 77–90.

Warren, K. 1997. Mayan self-determination: Multicultural models and educational choice for Guatemala. In W. Danspeckgrubery and A. Watts (eds.), *Self-Determination and Self-Administration: A Sourcebook*. Boulder, CO: Lynne Rienner Publisher, pp. 179–198.

Watts, J. 23 March 2013. Brazilian riot police evict Indigenous people near Rio's Maracanã stadium. *The Guardian*. Guardian News and Media. Available online at: http://www. theguardian.com/world/2013/mar/22/brazilian-police-evict-Indigenous-people

Weaver, H.N. 2012. Urban and Indigenous: The challenges of being a Native American in the city. *Journal of Community Practice* 20(4): 470–488.

Weber, M. 1978. *Economy and Society*. Berkeley, CA: University of California Press.

Weber-Pillwax, C. 2004. Indigenous researchers and Indigenous research methods: Cultural influences or cultural determinants of research methods. *Pimatisiwin: A Journal of Aboriginal and Indigenous Community Health* 2(1): 77–90.

Webster, S. 2000. The health and well-being of Aboriginal children and youth. In *The Health of Canada's Children: A CICH Profile*, 3rd edn. Ottawa: Canadian Institute of Child Health, pp. 143–172.

Welker, G. 2007. *Return to Indigenous Peoples' Literature*. Available online at: http:// www.Indigenouspeople.net [Accessed on 03 October 2007].

Wexler, L., White, J., and Trainor, B. 2015. Why an alternative to suicide prevention gatekeeper training is needed for rural Indigenous communities: presenting an empowering community storytelling approach. *Critical Public Health*. 25(2): 205–217.

Wherrett, J. 1999. *Aboriginal Self-Government*. Canada: Political and Social Affairs Division. Parliamentary Research Branch.

Wilkinson, R., and Marmot, M. (Eds.). 2003. *Social Determinants of Health: The Solid Facts*. Copenhagen: World Health Organization. Available online at: www.who.dk/document/ E81384.pdf

Williamson, J., and Dalal, P. 2007. Indigenising the curriculum or negotiating the tensions at the cultural interface? Embedding Indigenous perspectives and pedagogies in a university curriculum. *The Australian Journal of Indigenous Education* 36S: 51–58.

Wilson, K., and Young, T.K. 2008. An overview of Aboriginal health research in the social sciences: Current trends and future directions. *International Journal of Circumpolar Health* 67: 179–189.

Wong, Y.S., Allotey, P., and Reidpath, D.D. 2014. Health care as commons: An Indigenous approach to universal health coverage. *The International Indigenous Policy Journal* 5(3): 1–26.

World Bank. 7 June 1993. *Indigenous People in Latin America*. HRO Dissemination Notes. Human Resources Development and Operations Policy. Number 8. Washington: World Bank.

World Bank. 2000. *Ecuador: Crisis, Poverty and Social Services*. Washington: World Bank.

World Bank. July 2001. *Implementation of Operational Directive 4.20 on Indigenous Peoples: An Independent Desk Review Background Paper I. A Review of Selected Issues Related to IP*. Washington: OEDCR.

World Bank. 2013. *China: Poverty Alleviation through Community Participation*. Report. Washington: World Bank.

The World Bank Policy Brief. *Indigenous People: Still among the Poorest of the Poor*. Available online at: http://siteresources.worldbank.org/EXTINDPEOPLE/Resources/407801–1271860301656/HDNEN_Indigenous_clean_0421.pdf

World Health Organization (WHO). 1986. *Ottawa Charter for Health Promotion*. Geneva: World Heath Organization.

World Health Organization (WHO). 2006. *The Health of Indigenous People*. Geneva: World Heath Organization.

World Health Organization (WHO). October 2012. *What Is Universal Health Coverage?* Available online at: http://www.who.int/features/qa/universal_health_coverage/en/index.html

Xanthaki, A. 2002. Land rights of Indigenous people in South-East Asia. *Melbourne Journal of International Law* 4: 468.

Young, T.K. 2003. Review of research on Aboriginal populations in Canada: Relevance to their health needs. *British Medical Journal* 327: 419–422. doi:10.1136/bmj.327.7412.419

Young, T.K. 2006. *Practicing Self-Determination: Participation in Planning and Local Governance in Discrete Indigenous Settlements*. Unpublished PhD thesis, School of Geography, Planning and Architecture, University of Queensland, Brisbane.

Ling, Y.V., and Raphael, D. September/October 2004. Identifying and addressing the social determinants of the incidence and successful management of type 2 diabetes mellitus in Canada. *Canadian Journal of Public Health* 95(5): 366–68.

Zardo, M.N.L. 2013. Gender equality and Indigenous peoples' right to self-determination and culture. *American University International Law Review* 28(4): 1053–1090.

Zibechi, R. 2010. *Dispersing Power: Social Movements as Anti-State Forces*. Translated by Ramor Ryan. Oakland, CA: AK Press.

Zlotkin, N. 2009. From time immemorial: Recognition of Aboriginal customary law in Canada. In C. E. Bell, and R. K. Paterson (eds.), *Protection of First Nations Cultural Heritage: Laws, Policy, and Reform*. Vancouver: UBC Press, pp. 343–369.

Zoomers, A. 2008. Global traveling along the Inca Route: Is international tourism beneficial for local development? *European Planning Studies* 16(7): 971. Available at: ABI/INFORM Global database (Document ID: 1538585771). [Accessed on 10 March 2009].

Zubrick, S., Lawrence, D., Silburn, S., Blair, E., Milroy, H., Wilkes, T., Eades, S., et al. 2004. *The Western Australian Aboriginal Child Health Survey: The Health of Aboriginal Children and Young People*. Perth: Telethon Institute for Child Health Research.

Zubrick, S.R., D'Antoine, H., and the WAACHS Team. 2011. The mental health of Australian Aboriginal children and adolescents: Current status and future prospects. In H.E. Fitzgerald, K. Puura, M. Tomlinson, and P. Campbell (eds.), *International Perspectives on Children and Mental Health. Vol. 2: Prevention and Treatment*. Santa Barbara: CA: Praeger, pp. 155–183.

Zürcher, E. J. 2004. *Turkey: A Modern History*. London: I.B. Tauris.

Index